Deciphering
Difficult ECGs

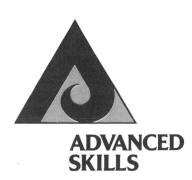

**ADVANCED
SKILLS**

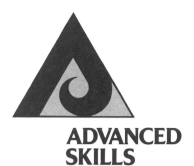

ADVANCED SKILLS

Deciphering Difficult ECGs

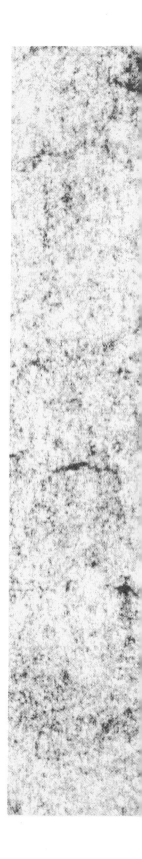

Springhouse Corporation
Springhouse, Pennsylvania

Staff

Executive Director, Editorial
Stanley Loeb

Editorial Director
Matthew Cahill

Clinical Director
Barbara F. McVan, RN

Art Director
John Hubbard

Senior Editor
William J. Kelly

Clinical Project Director
Patricia Dwyer Schull, RN, MSN

Editors
Stephen Daly, Elizabeth Weinstein, Marylou Ambrose, Jody Charnow, Catherine Harold, Elizabeth Mauro, Edith McMahon, Gale Sloan, Barbara Trenk, Jean Wallace

Clinical Editors
Tina R. Dietrich, RN, BSN, CCRN; Linda Roy, RN, MSN, CCRN; Brenda Salatino, RN, BSN, CCRN

Copy Editors
Jane V. Cray (supervisor), Christina A. Price, Nancy Papsin

Designers
Stephanie Peters (associate art director), Matie Patterson (senior designer), Lynn Foulk, Joseph Laufer

Illustrators
Kevin Curry, Jean Gardner, Linda Gist, Robert Jackson, Robert Neumann, Mary Stangl

Art Production
Robert Wieder

Typography
David Kosten (director), Diane Paluba (manager), Elizabeth Bergman, Joyce Rossi Biletz, Phyllis Marron, Robin Mayer, Valerie Rosenberger

Manufacturing
Deborah Meiris (manager), Anna Brindisi, T.A. Landis

Production Coordination
Colleen M. Hayman, Patricia W. McCloskey

Editorial Assistants
Maree DeRosa, Beverly Lane, Mary Madden, Margaret Rastiello

The clinical procedures described and recommended in this publication are based on research and consultation with nursing, medical, and legal authorities. To the best of our knowledge, these procedures reflect currently accepted practice; nevertheless, they can't be considered absolute and universal recommendations. For individual application, all recommendations must be considered in light of the patient's clinical condition and, before administration of new or infrequently used drugs, in light of the latest package-insert information. The authors and the publisher disclaim responsibility for any adverse effects resulting directly or indirectly from the suggested procedures, from any undetected errors, or from the reader's misunderstanding of the text.

Library of Congress Cataloging-in-Publication Data
Deciphering difficult ECGs.
        p.   cm. — (Advanced skills)
    Includes bibliographical references and index.
    1. Electrocardiography. 2. Heart — Diseases — Nursing.
I. Springhouse Corporation. II. Series.
    [DNLM: 1. Electrocardiography — methods — nurses' instruction. 2. Nursing Diagnosis — methods. WY 152.5 D294]
RC683.5.E5D34 1993
616.1'207547 — dc20
ONLM/DLC   92-49411
ISBN 0-87434-552-9   CIP

Contents

Advisory board vi
Contributors vii
Foreword viii

Part 1: Reviewing fundamentals
CHAPTER 1
Cardiac anatomy and physiology 3
Patti Hanisch, RN, MS, CCRN

Part 2: Interpreting rhythm strips
CHAPTER 2
Reading ECGs 17
Anne Marie H. Bularzik, RN, MSN

CHAPTER 3
Single-lead monitoring 31
Anne Marie H. Bularzik, RN, MSN

CHAPTER 4
Arrhythmia recognition 41
Barbara Leeper, RN, MN, CCRN

Part 3: Interpreting 12-lead ECGs
CHAPTER 5
Normal 12-lead ECG 67
Margaret A. Fitzgerald, RN,C, MS

CHAPTER 6
Electrical axis determination 79
Kathleen M. Hill, RN, MSN, CCRN

CHAPTER 7
Unstable angina 87
Sheila P. Leach, RN, MSN, CCRN, CS

CHAPTER 8
Acute myocardial infarction 97
Linda Roy, RN, MSN, CCRN

CHAPTER 9
Heart blocks 117
Myra Caplan, RN, MSN

CHAPTER 10
Tachycardias 133
Fred Langer, RN, BS

CHAPTER 11
Electrolyte disturbances 155
Lynn L. Cochran, RN, MS

Part 4: Understanding the effects of treatment
CHAPTER 12
Antiarrhythmic drugs 171
Flerida A. Imperial, RN, MN

CHAPTER 13
Pacemakers 191
Deborah Panozzo Nelson, RN, MS, CCRN

Suggested readings 210
Advanced skilltest 211
Index 224

Advisory board

At the time of publication, the advisors
held the following positions.

Cecelia Gatson Grindel, RN, PhD
Assistant Professor
Villanova University
College of Nursing
Villanova, Pa.

Judith Ski Lower, RN, MSN, CCRN, CNRN
Nurse Manager, Neurology Critical Care Unit
Johns Hopkins Hospital
Baltimore, Md.

Kathleen M. Malloch, RN, BSN, MBA, CNA
Clinical Nursing Administrator
Maryvale Samaritan Medical Center
Phoenix, Ariz.

Marguerite K. Schlag, RN, MSN, EdD
Director, Nursing Education and Development
Robert Wood Johnson University Hospital
New Brunswick, N.J.

Karen Then, RN, MN
Assistant Professor, Faculty of Nursing
University of Calgary, Alberta

Contributors

At the time of publication, the contributors
held the following positions.

Anne Marie H. Bularzik, RN, MSN

Director of Professional Development, Education
Holy Family Hospital and Medical Center
Methuen, Mass.

Myra Caplan, RN, MSN

Director of Staff Development
Kennedy Memorial Hospital–Stratford (N.J.)
Division

Lynn L. Cochran, RN, MS

Assistant Unit Leader, Clinical Specialist
Medical Intensive Care Unit, Rush-Presbyterian-
St. Luke's Medical Center
Chicago

Margaret A. Fitzgerald, RN,C, MS

Assistant Professor
Graduate School for Health Studies
Simmons College
Boston
Family Nurse Practitioner
The Family Health Center
Lawrence, Mass.

Patti Hanisch, RN, MS, CCRN

Nursing Instructor, Cardiac Rehabilitation
Coordinator
Royal C. Johnson Veterans Affairs Medical Center
Sioux Falls, S.D.

Kathleen M. Hill, RN, MSN, CCRN

Clinical Nurse Specialist, Intensive Care Unit
Lakewood (Ohio) Hospital

Flerida A. Imperial, RN, MN

Clinical Nurse Specialist, Cardiothoracic Intensive
Care Unit
UCLA Medical Center
Los Angeles

Fred Langer, RN, BS

Critical Care Educator (Cardiovascular)
Florida Hospital Medical Center
Orlando

Sheila P. Leach, RN, MSN, CCRN, CS

Clinical Nurse Manager, Cardiovascular
Surgical Unit
Western Reserve Care System
Youngstown, Ohio

Barbara Leeper, RN, MN, CCRN

Cardiovascular Clinical Nurse Specialist
Baylor University Medical Center
Dallas

Deborah Panozzo Nelson, RN, MS, CCRN

Cardiovascular Clinical Specialist
EMS Nursing Education
LaGrange, Ill.
Adjunct Faculty
Lewis University
Romeoville, Ill.

Linda Roy, RN, MSN, CCRN

Clinical Instructor, Critical Care
Doylestown (Pa.) Hospital

FOREWORD

Electrocardiogram (ECG) monitors and machines are no longer confined to critical care units. Today, no matter where you work or what your specialty, you need to know how to read an ECG.

But interpreting an ECG—especially a difficult one—requires special knowledge and skill. You need to understand not only the fundamentals of electrocardiography but also how to recognize various arrhythmias on a rhythm strip and how to identify disorders, such as heart blocks, unstable angina, and myocardial infarction, on a 12-lead ECG.

Fortunately, *Deciphering Difficult ECGs* provides you with all you need to interpret even the most puzzling waveforms. By reading this book and practicing the skills it teaches, you'll become more and more proficient at interpreting complex ECGs.

This book consists of four parts. The first one, "Reviewing fundamentals," presents an overview of basic principles you must understand before interpreting difficult ECGs. Here you'll find clear, concise explanations of cardiac anatomy and physiology, and the mechanisms that trigger arrhythmias. To facilitate your review of these topics, this section also contains four pages of color illustrations showing cardiac anatomy, the conduction system, and circus reentry.

The next part, which contains three chapters, focuses on interpreting rhythm strips. Chapter 2 provides brief explanations of electrocardiography, leads and planes, and the components of the ECG waveform. Chapter 3 details single-lead monitoring—both hardwire and telemetry—and explains how such monitoring can help you evaluate a patient's ongoing cardiac rhythm. Chapter 4 focuses on how to recognize about 20 of the most common arrhythmias. For your convenience, each arrhythmia is covered on a single page that includes an ECG strip, ECG characteristics and interpretation, a general description, assessment findings, and interventions.

The third part—the heart of *Deciphering Difficult ECGs*—covers how to interpret 12-lead ECGs. Chapter 5 explains how to set up and use a 12-lead ECG machine. In this chapter, you'll find a 3-page photoguide showing you exactly how to record 12-lead ECGs. Then chapter 6 provides an easy-to-understand explanation of a difficult topic—axis determination.

The next five chapters explain and depict how to identify cardiac disorders using a 12-lead ECG. Chapter 7 covers unstable angina; chapter 8, acute myocardial infarction; chapter 9, heart blocks; chapter 10, tachycardia; and chapter 11, electrolyte disturbances. In each of these chapters, you'll find 12-lead ECGs that show key characteristics of various disorders. For instance, in chapter 9, you'll find 12-lead ECGs showing right bundle-branch block, left bundle-branch block, left anterior hemiblock, left posterior hemiblock, and both types of bifascicular block. For your convenience and easy reference, the leads showing diagnostic ECG changes are graphically highlighted on every 12-lead ECG in the book.

The book's final part discusses the effects of treatment on ECGs. Chapter 12 covers the effects of antiarrhythmic drugs; chapter 13, the effects of pacemakers.

Throughout the book, you'll see graphic devices called logos that direct you to essential information. The *Lead of choice* logo signals an explanation of which lead you should use to monitor a patient with a particular condition. For example, the *Lead of choice* on page 144 explains that you should use lead II to monitor a patient with narrow QRS-complex tachycardia. It also includes lead II rhythm strips for four different types of narrow QRS-complex tachycardia.

With each *Pathophysiology* logo, you'll find an illustration and explanation of the underlying cause of a cardiac disorder. The *Troubleshooting* logo signals information on how to identify and correct an equipment problem.

Following the last chapter is a listing of suggested readings. Then comes an *Advanced skilltest,* created to help you test your knowledge of ECG interpretation. This test contains

cases histories, rhythm strips, and 12-lead ECGs as well as answers with rationales.

Deciphering Difficult ECGs is designed for all nurses who must meet the challenge of interpreting their patients' ECGs. With its straightforward writing and its many helpful features, this book is simply a must for any working nurse. I strongly recommend it.

Brenda Salatino, RN, BSN, CCRN
Consultant
Bethlehem, Pa

PART 1

Reviewing fundamentals

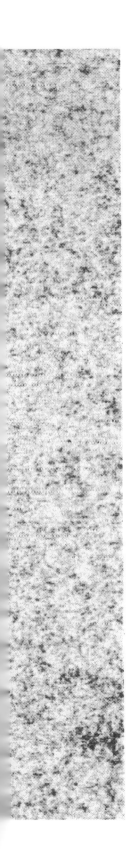

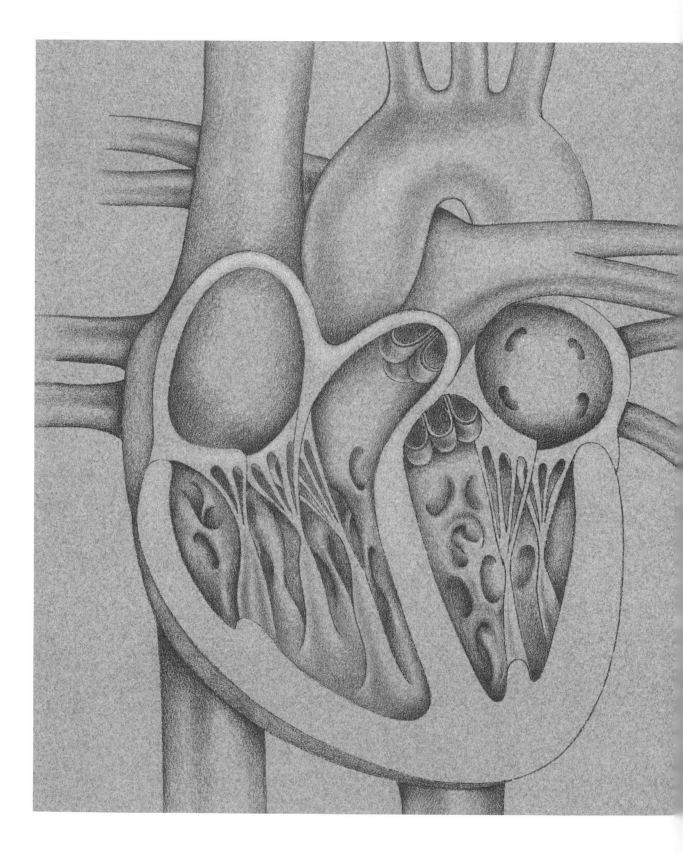

CHAPTER

1

Cardiac anatomy and physiology

Today, patients with cardiovascular problems are no longer cared for exclusively in intensive care or critical care units. Within days after admission to these units, the patients may be transferred to a medical-surgical unit and then to an extended care facility. As a result, nurses in widely varied settings must provide thorough, efficient cardiovascular care. And one of the most essential—and sophisticated—skills you need to provide such care is interpreting electrocardiograms (ECGs).

This chapter lays the groundwork for reading both rhythm strips and 12-lead ECGs by concisely reviewing cardiac anatomy and physiology. The first part of the chapter covers the heart's location, structure, and blood supply. Next comes a discussion of the conduction system and electrophysiology. Finally, you'll find a brief discussion of the mechanisms that cause cardiac arrhythmias.

Anatomy

The center of the cardiovascular system, the heart delivers oxygenated blood throughout the body via the arteries. A normal adult heart contracts at a rate of 60 to 100 beats/minute, pumping 5.5 liters of blood/minute over 60,000 miles of blood vessels.

Location and structure

The heart lies in the mediastinum, the mass of tissue between the lungs that extends from the sternum to the spine. About two-thirds of the heart extends to the left of the body's midline. The bottom of the heart, or the apex, tilts forward and down toward the left side of the body and rests on the diaphragm. The top of the heart, or the base, lies just below the second rib. (See *The heart's location*.)

A hollow, cone-shaped, muscular organ roughly the size of a fist, the heart is about 5" (12 cm) long and 3½" (9 cm) wide. It weighs between 9 and 12 oz (250 and 350 g), depending on a person's age, sex, and body size. In athletic young people, the heart may weigh slightly more than 12 oz; in elderly people, it may weigh slightly less than 9 oz.

Heart wall

A three-part wall surrounds the heart, and a thick fibrous sac, the pericardium, holds it in place. The inner layer, or endocardium, consists of a thin layer of endothelial tissue that lines the heart valves and chambers. The myocardium, the middle and thickest layer, consists of the muscle that contracts with each heartbeat. The outermost layer, the epicardium, forms the inner layer of the pericardium, which envelops the heart and contains pericardial fluid that lubricates and protects the heart from friction.

This inner layer of the pericardium is also known as the visceral layer of the serous pericardium. It contains the main coronary vessels, as well as the autonomic nerves, lymphatic channels, and fatty tissue. Between the visceral layer and the parietal layer of the serous pericardium is a thin film of serous fluid that holds the layers together, much as a thin film of

water holds two microscope slides. The outside layer of the pericardium is known as the fibrous pericardium. (See *Layers of the heart wall*, page 7.)

Cardiac chambers

The heart has four chambers—two atria and two ventricles. The atria act as collectors for the ventricles, which produce the heart's pumping action. The right side of the heart receives blood from the systemic veins and propels it to the lungs for oxygen supply and carbon dioxide removal. The left side of the heart receives oxygenated blood from the pulmonary veins and pumps it into the systemic circulation. The interatrial septum separates the right and left atria; the interventricular septum separates the right and left ventricles.

The thickness of the walls in each chamber corresponds to the degree of high-pressure work performed by that chamber. Because the atria serve as reservoirs and conduits for blood funneled into the ventricles, their walls are relatively thin. The left ventricle has much thicker walls than the right ventricle because it must pump blood through the systemic circulation. (See *Inside view of a normal heart*, page 7.)

Valves

Four cardiac valves keep the blood flowing through the heart in the right direction. The opening and closing of these valves depend on pressure gradients on both sides of them.

The two atrioventricular (AV) valves separate the atria from the ventricles, preventing a backflow of blood during ventricular contraction. The tricuspid valve, which has three triangular cusps, controls blood flow between the right atrium and the right ventricle. The mitral or bicuspid valve separates the left atrium from the left ventricle. Strong filaments called chordae tendineae attach the cusps of these valves to the ventricles' papillary muscles. The chordae tendineae and the papillary muscles stabilize the valves and prevent valve leaflet eversion. A dysfunction of the chordae tendineae or papillary muscles can cause an incomplete closure of an AV valve, resulting in a murmur.

Known as the semilunar valves, the pulmonary and aortic valves each have three cuplike

The heart's location

The heart lies within the mediastinum, as shown. Note that two-thirds of the heart extends to the left of the body's midline.

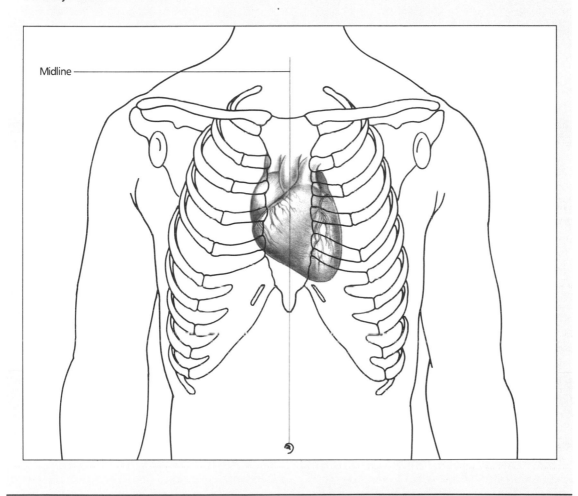

Midline

cusps. These valves open and close passively, responding to pressure changes caused by ventricular contraction and blood ejection. The pulmonary valve separates the right ventricle from the pulmonary artery. The aortic valve allows blood to flow from the left ventricle to the aorta. The closing of these valves prevents a backflow of blood into the ventricles.

Heart's blood supply

Because it continuously pumps blood throughout the body, the heart demands a constant and reliable source of oxygen. The coronary arteries and their branches supply the heart with oxygenated blood and metabolic substrates, while the cardiac veins remove carbon dioxide and other wastes.

When the heart's metabolic demands increase, coronary blood flow can increase to more than five times its resting amount. Because myocardial oxygen extraction stays fixed at about 65% to 70% of stroke volume regardless of physiologic condition, enhanced coronary blood flow is the heart's only way of meeting its increased oxygen needs.

Coronary arteries

The right coronary artery and the left main coronary artery originate as a single branch of the ascending aorta. The right coronary artery supplies blood to the right atrium, right ventricle, and part of the inferior and posterior surfaces of the left ventricle. In most people, the right coronary artery supplies the sinoatrial (SA) node; in others, the circumflex artery supplies most of the blood to the SA node. The right coronary artery also supplies blood to the bundle of His and to the AV node. (See *Vessels of the heart,* page 8.)

The left main coronary artery runs over the surface of the left atrium, where it divides into two major branches: the left anterior descending (LAD) artery and the left circumflex artery. The LAD artery descends toward the heart's apex. With its branches, the diagonal arteries and septal perforators, the LAD artery supplies blood to the walls of both ventricles. The circumflex artery distributes oxygenated blood to the walls of the left ventricle and left atrium.

The right coronary artery is often called the dominant artery—even though in most people, it is narrower and perfuses less of the myocardium than the left main coronary artery. The reason: The artery that crosses the crux (the point where the right and left AV grooves cross the posterior interatrial and interventricular grooves) is always referred to as the dominant artery. And, in most people, that vessel is the right coronary artery.

Coronary artery blood flow

During ventricular systole, the coronary arteries are squeezed, impeding blood flow. So the coronary arteries receive blood primarily during ventricular diastole, when the aortic valve closes. Whatever shortens the diastolic time, then, such as tachycardia, will diminish coronary artery blood flow. During bradycardia, diastole is prolonged, but coronary flow may

be impeded by a lack of adequate pressure and aortic recoil.

Cardiac veins

The thebesian veins, the anterior cardiac veins, and the coronary sinus and its tributaries drain blood from the myocardium into the right atrium. These cardiac veins run parallel to the coronary arteries.

Collateral circulation

When two or more arteries supply the same region, they usually connect with each other via anastomoses within the myocardium. These anastomoses provide collateral circulation, or alternate blood routes. Typically, the myocardium contains numerous anastomoses connecting the branches of the coronary arteries.

Collateral arteries may be present at birth, but they usually develop when oxygen demands change. Conditions such as coronary artery disease, chronic myocardial hypoxia, and myocardial hypertrophy can cause collateral circulation to develop. Although most collateral arteries in the heart are small, heart muscle can remain alive as long as it receives 10% to 15% of its normal blood supply.

Physiology

The heart pumps blood by muscular contraction—a function that depends on the interaction between an electrical stimulus and a mechanical response. Correct interpretation of an ECG—which represents the heart's electrical activity—depends on an understanding of how the conduction system carries electrical impulses through the heart and how electrical activity occurs in myocardial cells.

Conduction system

For a contraction to take place, the heart must conduct impulses via a specialized route. This route consists of the SA node, internodal tracts and Bachmann's bundle, AV node, bundle of

(Text continues on page 11.)

Inside view of a normal heart

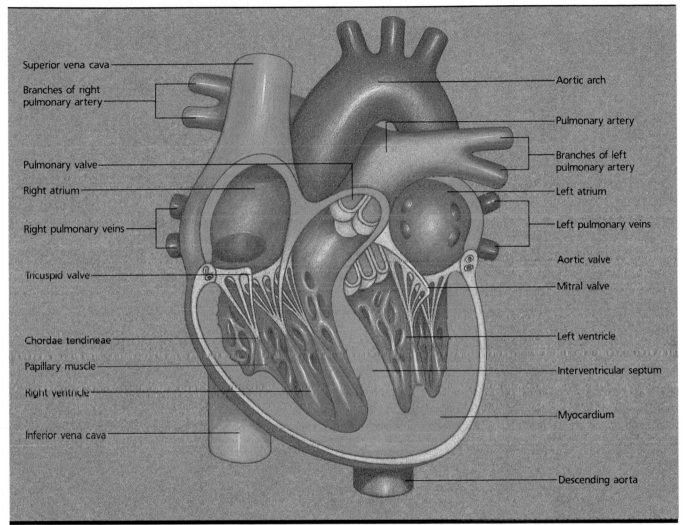

Superior vena cava
Branches of right pulmonary artery
Pulmonary valve
Right atrium
Right pulmonary veins
Tricuspid valve
Chordae tendineae
Papillary muscle
Right ventricle
Inferior vena cava

Aortic arch
Pulmonary artery
Branches of left pulmonary artery
Left atrium
Left pulmonary veins
Aortic valve
Mitral valve
Left ventricle
Interventricular septum
Myocardium
Descending aorta

Layers of the heart wall

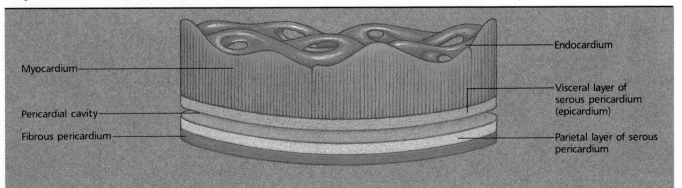

Myocardium
Pericardial cavity
Fibrous pericardium

Endocardium
Visceral layer of serous pericardium (epicardium)
Parietal layer of serous pericardium

Vessels of the heart

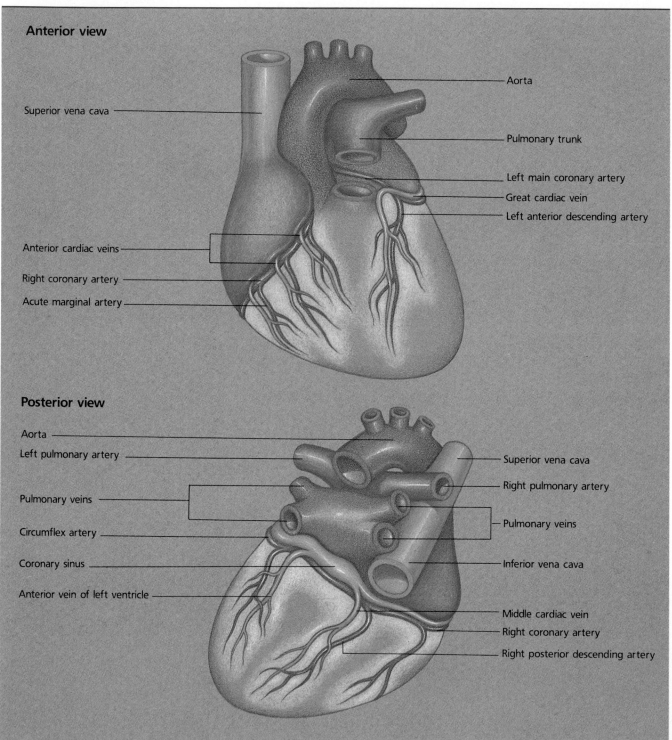

Anterior view

Superior vena cava

Aorta

Pulmonary trunk

Left main coronary artery

Great cardiac vein

Left anterior descending artery

Anterior cardiac veins

Right coronary artery

Acute marginal artery

Posterior view

Aorta

Left pulmonary artery

Pulmonary veins

Circumflex artery

Coronary sinus

Anterior vein of left ventricle

Superior vena cava

Right pulmonary artery

Pulmonary veins

Inferior vena cava

Middle cardiac vein

Right coronary artery

Right posterior descending artery

Conduction system

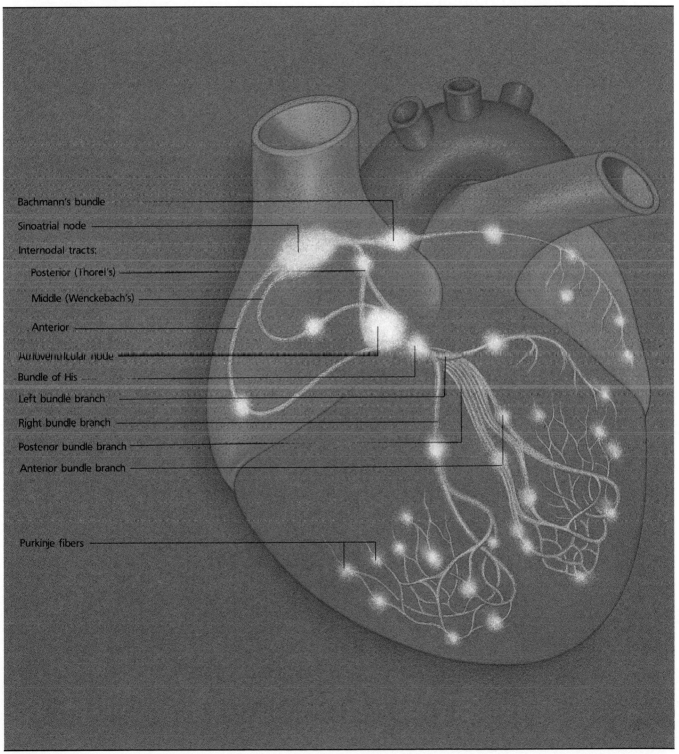

Bachmann's bundle

Sinoatrial node

Internodal tracts:

    Posterior (Thorel's)

    Middle (Wenckebach's)

    Anterior

Atrioventricular node

Bundle of His

Left bundle branch

Right bundle branch

Posterior bundle branch

Anterior bundle branch

Purkinje fibers

Understanding circus reentry

For circus reentry to develop, the following conditions are necessary:
• An initiating impulse—either a normal sinus impulse or an ectopic impulse—must be present.
• An area of conduction must slow the impulse so it's still active when the surrounding myocardium repolarizes.
• Unidirectional conduction must occur, preventing the impulse from neutralizing itself in the area of slow conduction.

The illustrations on this page show impulse transmission through a loop in a conduction pathway.

Bidirectional conduction
The first set of illustrations shows two separate events. In each, conduction occurs in two directions, so circuit reentry can't occur.

An impulse travels down a pathway, splits in two directions, and meets in the lower common pathway.

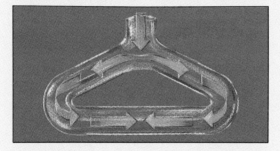

Again, the impulse moves down the initial pathway. After being blocked in the left branch, it's quickly transmitted down the right branch and back up to the block. Here the impulse is cancelled because the area remains refractory. The two-way conduction and fast transmission prevent circus reentry.

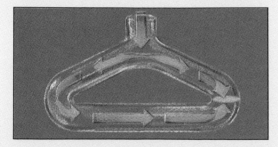

Unidirectional conduction
The following set of illustrations shows a sequence in which an impulse is conducted in only one direction, making circus reentry possible.

A block in the left branch stops the impulse, which is then slowly conducted down the right branch and into the common pathway.

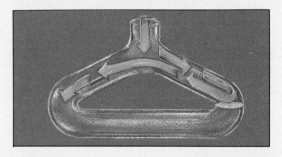

Still traveling slowly, the impulse reaches the block. In the time it takes to get there, the cardiac tissue has become repolarized, so the impulse can enter the block on the left.

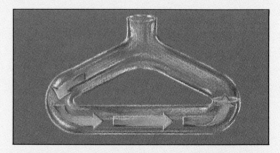

Circus reentry occurs as the impulse reenters the initial pathway and the right branch.

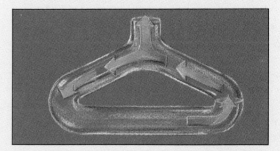

His, bundle branches, and Purkinje fibers. (See *Conduction system,* page 9.)

SA node

The cardiac rhythm normally originates in the SA node—located where the superior vena cava enters the right atrium. Acting as the heart's main pacemaker, the SA node initiates 60 to 100 beats/minute under resting conditions.

Internodal tracts and Bachmann's bundle

How impulses travel from the SA node through the right atrium is uncertain. According to one theory, the impulse is transmitted through the right atrium via three internodal tracts: the anterior, the middle (Wenckebach's), and the posterior (Thorel's). However, the existence of these tracts is a matter of debate among researchers.

The impulse travels to the left atrium via Bachmann's bundle. This transmission occurs so quickly that the left atrium contracts almost simultaneously with the right atrium.

AV node

After traversing the atria, an impulse arrives at the AV node located in the inferior right atrium near the ostium of the coronary sinus. The AV node delays the impulse by 0.04 second, giving the ventricles a chance to fill with blood while the atria contract. The AV node can't generate a spontaneous impulse, but the junctional tissue around it can.

Bundle of His

Following the 0.04-second delay in the AV node, an impulse rapidly moves through the bundle of His—the beginning of the ventricular conduction system. The bundle of His divides into the right and left bundle branches.

A pacemaker site, the bundle of His has an intrinsic firing rate between 40 and 60 beats/ minute. Usually the bundle of His fires when the SA node doesn't generate an impulse at a normal rate, or when the impulse doesn't reach the AV node.

Bundle branches

Conduction continues through the right and left bundle branches, which extend down either side of the interventricular septum. Thicker than the right bundle branch, the left bundle branch divides into two fascicles. Conduction velocity in the left bundle branch exceeds that in the right, giving the larger muscle of the left ventricle the extra time needed to contract at the same time as the right ventricle.

Purkinje fibers

After traveling down the bundle branches, an impulse enters the peripheral Purkinje system, which covers the endocardial surfaces of both ventricles. The impulse spreads from the endocardium to the ventricular myocardium and epicardium.

Another pacemaker site, the Purkinje fibers normally fire when higher pacemakers fail to generate an impulse, or when the impulse is blocked at or above the bundle branches. The automatic firing rate of the Purkinje fibers ranges from 15 to 40 beats/minute.

Escape rhythms

An escape rhythm may be precipitated by an escape beat, which is a compensatory mechanism that originates in the AV junction or the ventricles. An escape beat occurs when a higher pacemaker site fails to fire, or its rate of firing slows, and the next pacemaker site in the conduction sequence takes over. Common escape rhythms that may result include idioventricular, accelerated idioventricular, and junctional rhythms.

Electrophysiology

Electrical impulses are transmitted through the heart's conduction system to create rhythmic contractions. But what initiates the electrical events? The cyclic exchange of sodium, potassium, and calcium across myocardial cell membranes results in electrical depolarization and repolarization of the cells. Any disruption in this cycle will cause a change in the electrical forces needed to maintain normal rhythmic contractions.

Membrane potential

Electrical activity can be generated in myocardial cells because they have a membrane potential—that is, a potential for electrical activity created by a semipermeable membrane that allows the passage of sodium, potassium, and calcium ions. The cycle of ion shifts continuously changes the electrical charge inside the cells, causing periods of rest (or repolarization) and periods of activity (depolarization). Actually, there are two types of membrane potentials that allow these periods of rest and activity: the resting membrane potential and the action potential.

Resting membrane potential

The resting membrane potential occurs when the electrical charge inside the cell is more negative than the charge outside the cell. The intracellular charge becomes more negative because the cell membrane is more permeable to potassium than to sodium. Thus, potassium easily moves out of the cell, but sodium doesn't move in as readily. The relatively lower intracellular concentration creates the negative charge.

In this resting state, the cells are said to be polarized and no electrical activity occurs in them. This stage is represented on an ECG by an isoelectric line.

Action potential

When a sufficient stimulus occurs—either from a neighboring cell or from a pacemaker cell—the membrane permeability changes. A resulting exchange of ions across the membrane makes the intracellular charge less negative than the extracellular charge. This causes an action potential or cell depolarization.

Nonpacemaker cells have a property known as excitability, which allows them to respond to a stimulus. These cells are excitable because of their instability, a result of the constant ion traffic across their membranes. Pacemaker cells, however, have a property called automaticity, which allows them to initiate an impulse spontaneously or to propagate an action potential.

Phases of depolarization-repolarization

The complete cycle of cellular action and rest (or depolarization and repolarization) is usually divided into five phases, numbered 0 through 4. (See *Five phases of depolarization and repolarization,* opposite, and *Action potential curve,* page 14.)

Phase 0

The period of rapid depolarization, phase 0 begins when the cell membrane is stimulated and suddenly becomes permeable to sodium. At that point, sodium rapidly flows into the cell, and calcium trickles in. This changes the electrical charge of the cell from negative to positive. During depolarization, the calcium moving into the cell stimulates an attraction between the two muscle filaments, actin and myosin, triggering myocardial contraction.

Phase 1

After the rapid influx of sodium, a brief period of partial repolarization occurs, known as phase 1. Sodium stops flowing into the cell, and the electrical charge becomes more negative. The precise mechanism that causes phase 1 isn't understood.

Phase 2

During phase 2, or the plateau phase, about the same amount of calcium enters the cell as potassium leaves it. The cell is now supersaturated with ions.

Taken together, phase 1, phase 2, and the first part of phase 3 are known as the absolute or effective refractory period. The cell can't accept any stimulus at this point—no matter how strong. (See *Understanding refractory periods,* page 15.)

Phase 3

Known as the rapid repolarization phase, phase 3 depends on two processes. Calcium and sodium stop entering the cell, and large amounts of potassium exit the cell. Together these processes make the cell more negative. During the last half of phase 3—also known as the relative refractory period—the cell can respond only to a stimulus that's stronger than normal.

Five phases of depolarization and repolarization

Use this illustration to review the five phases of the heart's depolarization-repolarization cycle.

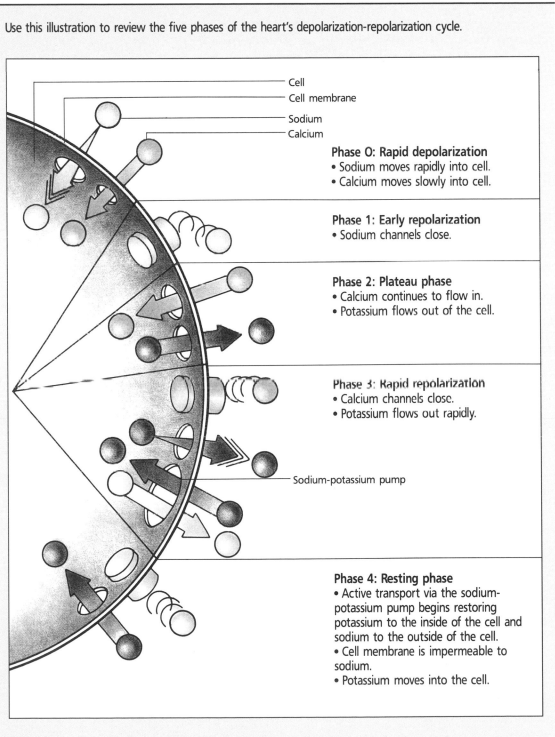

Cell
Cell membrane
Sodium
Calcium

Phase 0: Rapid depolarization
• Sodium moves rapidly into cell.
• Calcium moves slowly into cell.

Phase 1: Early repolarization
• Sodium channels close.

Phase 2: Plateau phase
• Calcium continues to flow in.
• Potassium flows out of the cell.

Phase 3: Rapid repolarization
• Calcium channels close.
• Potassium flows out rapidly.

Sodium-potassium pump

Phase 4: Resting phase
• Active transport via the sodium-potassium pump begins restoring potassium to the inside of the cell and sodium to the outside of the cell.
• Cell membrane is impermeable to sodium.
• Potassium moves into the cell.

Action potential curve

An action potential curve shows the electrical changes in myocardial cells during the depolarization-repolarization cycle. This graph shows the changes in a nonpacemaker cell.

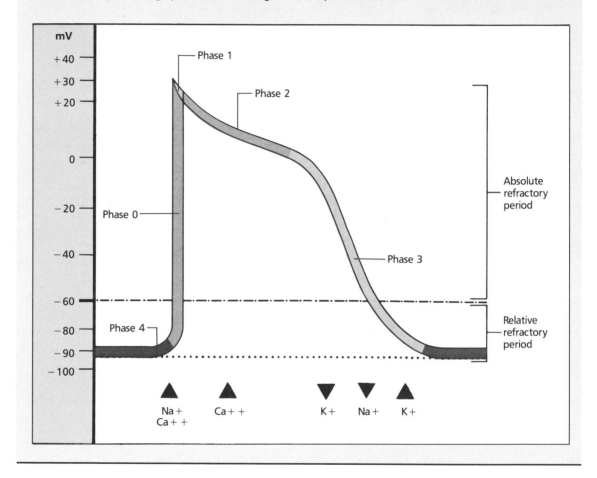

Phase 4

During phase 4, known as the resting phase, adenosine triphosphate activates the sodium-potassium pump, which removes the excess sodium that entered the cell during depolarization and moves potassium into the cell. This mechanism returns the intracellular concentrations of sodium and potassium to pre-depolarization levels. By the end of phase 4, the cell can receive an electrical stimulus once again.

Understanding arrhythmias

Now that you've reviewed how the heart generates normal rhythms, take a few minutes to read about the mechanisms that can cause cardiac arrhythmias: altered automaticity, retrograde conduction, reentry, and a phenomenon commonly called afterpotentials or after-depolarization and triggered activity.

Altered automaticity

Automaticity is a special characteristic of cardiac pacemaker cells, and when it either increases or decreases, an arrhythmia can result.

If phase 4 depolarization accelerates in the pacemaker cells below the SA node, automaticity will increase—possibly resulting in premature beats or tachycardia. This acceleration may have a variety of causes, including hypoxia, hypokalemia, hypocalcemia, hypercapnia, stretching of conductive fibers, elevated room temperature or hot weather, and trauma.

If the rate of spontaneous depolarization of the SA node decreases, bradycardia or escape rhythms may result. This deceleration may result from vagal stimulation, ischemia, hypothermia, a sudden rise in local extracellular potassium, or abnormally low catecholamine levels.

Retrograde conduction

When an electrical impulse is initiated at or below the AV node, it may be transmitted backward toward the atria. In this case, the propagation time is usually longer than with antegrade (or normal) conduction. The resulting arrhythmia disrupts the normal coordinated functions of the atria and ventricles.

Reentry

Reentry occurs when cardiac tissue is activated two or more times by the same impulse. Circus reentry takes place when conduction slows down, focal reentry when the refractory periods for neighboring cells don't coincide.

In circus reentry, an impulse is delayed in a slow conduction pathway and remains active when the surrounding myocardium repolarizes. The impulse then reenters the surrounding tissue, producing another impulse. (See *Understanding circus reentry,* page 10.)

In focal reentry, repolarizing cells reexcite cells that are already repolarized. This occurs when neighboring cells are activated at or about the same time, but repolarize at different rates. The result is a second impulse.

Understanding refractory periods

Normally, an impulse initiates an action potential at the end of phase 4—when a myocardial cell is completely polarized. But sometimes an impulse reaches a cell when it's still repolarizing. Can the cell accept the stimulus? That depends on the stage of repolarization.

During phases 1 and 2 and the first half of phase 3, known collectively as the absolute refractory period, or the effective refractory period, the cell can't be depolarized.

By the second half of phase 3, however, the cell starts becoming responsive. During this relative refractory (or vulnerable) period, a strong stimulus—or a normal one with delayed conduction—can initiate an action potential.

Afterdepolarization and triggered activity

In injured pacemaker or nonpacemaker cells, partial depolarization may occur. This can lead to spontaneous (secondary) depolarization—a repetitive ectopic firing called triggered activity. The depolarization produced by this triggered activity is known as afterdepolarization.

Early afterdepolarization occurs before the cell fully repolarizes. This phenomenon may result from hypokalemia, slow pacing rates, or drug toxicity. Delayed afterdepolarizations are small depolarizations (about 10 millivolts) that occur after the cells have repolarized. They are usually too small to reach the threshold voltage for triggering a contraction. But as the heart rate increases, or stimulation becomes more premature, the delayed afterdepolarization becomes larger and larger until the threshold voltage is reached and a run of rapid firing or triggered activity is reached. Factors increasing the amplitude of delayed afterdepolarization include elevated calcium levels, increased catecholamine concentration, and digitalis toxicity. Either atrial or ventricular tachycardia may be triggered by afterdepolarizations.

PART 2

Interpreting rhythm strips

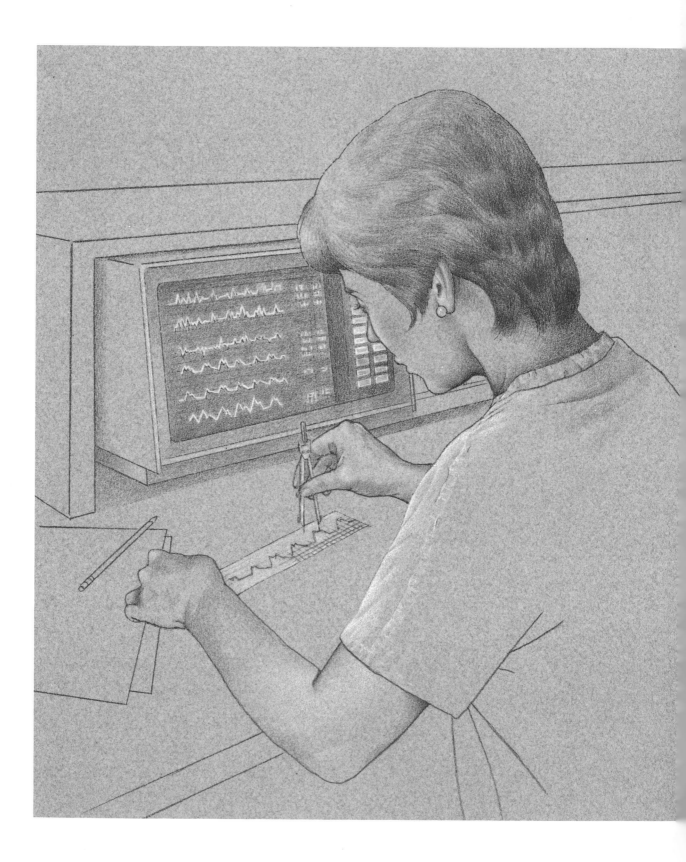

2

CHAPTER

Reading ECGs

Electrocardiography provides you with a graphic recording of the heart's electrical activity. In fact, each component of an electrocardiogram (ECG) or waveform represents a specific event in the depolarization-repolarization cycle. Thus, by interpreting an ECG correctly, you can identify rhythm and conduction disturbances and obtain other valuable information about your patient's cardiac status.

This chapter presents the essential information you need to interpret an ECG. After a brief review of electrocardiography, the chapter fully explains the individual components of a waveform. The chapter then concludes by presenting a systematic approach to analyzing an ECG.

Identifying waveform deflections

The direction of the electrical current determines the deflection of the electrocardiogram waveform. When the current travels toward the positive pole, the waveform deflects upward, as shown on the right. When the current travels toward the negative pole, the waveform deflects downward, as shown on the left. When the current flows perpendicular to the lead, the waveform may go in both directions, as shown at the top. The other two waveforms shown represent a current running at a 45-degree angle to the negative pole and a current running at a 45-degree angle to the positive pole.

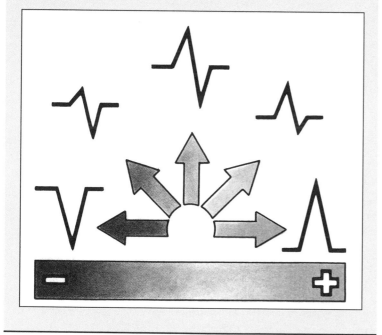

Electrocardiography

The heart's electrical activity generates currents that spread to the skin. Electrodes attached to the skin can pick up these currents and transmit them to an ECG machine. In the machine, the currents are transformed into waveforms representing the heart's depolarization-repolarization cycle. By studying these waveforms, you can see the precise sequence of electrical events occurring in your patient's heart.

Leads and planes

Created by either one or two electrodes, a lead provides you with a particular view of the electrical activity between two points, or poles. Every lead consists of a positive (+) pole and a negative (−) pole. Between the positive and negative poles is a line of sight, an imaginary line representing the lead's axis. When you look at a waveform, you see a deflection of the electrical current flowing between the two poles. Its direction will depend on the direction of the electrical current in relation to the axis. (See *Identifying waveform deflections*.)

If the current in the heart flows along the axis toward the positive pole, the waveform deflects upward and is referred to as a positive deflection. When the current flows along the axis away from the positive pole, the waveform deflects downward—a negative deflection. A current flowing perpendicular to the axis produces either very small waveforms or waveforms that go in two directions, called biphasic waveforms. When electrical activity is absent or too small to measure, the waveform is a straight line, called an isoelectric deflection.

A cross-section of the heart, a plane provides a different perspective of the heart's electrical activity. In the frontal plane—a vertical cut through the middle of the heart from top to bottom—electrical activity is viewed from superior to inferior. In the horizontal plane—a transverse cut through the middle of the heart—electrical activity is viewed from anterior to posterior.

Twelve leads
A complete picture of the heart's electrical activity consists of 12 leads—that is, 12 different views. But when you monitor a patient's heart rhythm, you'll usually look at one of these leads, typically lead II.

These 12 leads are divided into limb leads and precordial leads, based on the placement of the electrodes. The six limb leads, which re-

Examining the ECG grid

The increments on this sample electrocardiogram (ECG) grid let you determine the timing (horizontal axis) and amplitude (vertical axis) of waveforms. On the horizontal axis, a small block equals 0.04 second; five small blocks, 0.2 second; and five large blocks, 1 second. On the vertical axis, a small block equals 0.1 mV; a large block, 0.5 mV; and two large blocks, 1 mV.

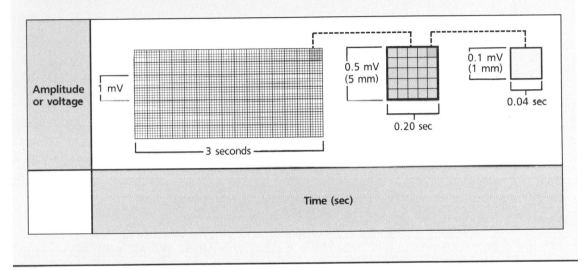

flect activity in the frontal plane, are leads I, II, III, aV$_R$ (augmented vector right), aV$_L$ (augmented vector left), and aV$_F$ (augmented vector foot). The six precordial leads, which reflect the horizontal plane, are called leads V$_1$, V$_2$, V$_3$, V$_4$, V$_5$, and V$_6$.

ECG strip

ECGs are recorded on heat-sensitive, standardized grid paper, using a heated stylus that moves at a normal speed of 25 mm/second.

The paper consists of a series of intersecting horizontal and vertical lines. The lines form small blocks, each 1 mm wide and 1 mm high. Horizontal lines represent time and vertical lines represent amplitude or voltage. (See *Examining the ECG grid*.)

When you measure the duration of a waveform, each small block on the horizontal axis (shown by the light lines) equals 0.04 second. Five small blocks form the base of a large block (shown by the heavy lines), which represents 0.20 second. So five large blocks equal 1 second. You can determine the duration by counting the number of small blocks from the beginning of the waveform to the end. Multiply that number by 0.04 second.

The speed of the recording stylus determines the time measurement. When you need to closely examine a particular aspect of the ECG, you can increase the speed from 25 mm/second to 50 mm/second. This spreads out the waveforms so you can differentiate certain arrhythmias.

On the vertical axis, amplitude or voltage is measured in millivolts (mV). Each small block represents 0.1 mV; each large block represents 0.5 mV. To measure the amplitude of a waveform, count the number of small blocks from the waveform base to its height and convert that into millimeters (mm). One millivolt equals 10 mm.

When the height of a waveform exceeds the size of the ECG paper, you may need to

Identifying ECG components

This strip shows the components of a normal electrocardiogram (ECG) waveform.

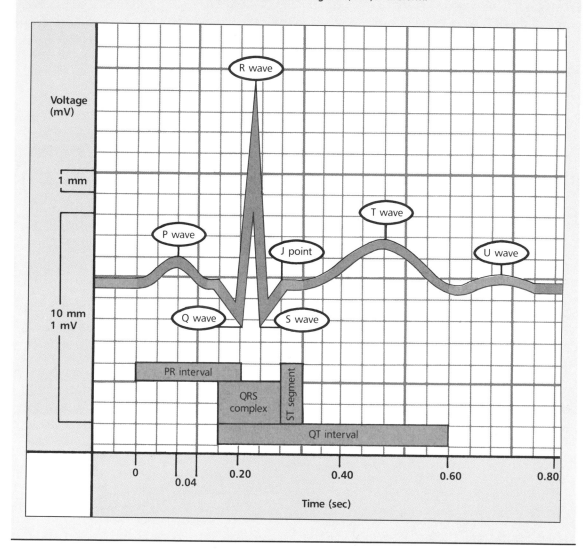

adjust the calibration standard by half. Similarly, you can double the standard when the waveform height is too small. In either case, remember the adjustment you've made when counting blocks to determine voltage.

ECG components

A normal ECG waveform has these components: the P wave, the PR interval, the QRS complex, the J point, the ST segment, the T wave, the QT interval and, in some cases, the Tp wave and the U wave. While the letters themselves have no special significance, each component represents a particular event in the depolarization-repolarization cycle. (See *Identifying ECG components*.)

P wave

The first component of a normal ECG waveform, the P wave represents atrial depolarization—the conduction of an electrical impulse through the atria. A normal P wave has the following characteristics:
• *Location*. Precedes the QRS complex.
• *Configuration*. Rounded and smooth, not pointed or notched.
• *Amplitude*. 2 to 3 mm.
• *Duration*. 0.06 to 0.12 second.
• *Deflection*. Upright in leads I, II, aV_F, V_2, V_3, V_4, V_5, and V_6. Usually positive but may be biphasic or inverted in leads III, aV_L, and V_1. Inverted in aV_R.

Significance
A normal P wave usually means the stimulus began in the sinoatrial (SA) node. An ECG shows the heart's depolarization and repolarization, but it can't show the actual firing of the SA node. That initial impulse produces no obvious deflection.

If a P wave precedes each QRS complex, the impulses are being conducted from the atria to the ventricles. Partway through the inscribing of the P wave, the atria start to contract. But this won't be evident from the ECG because it only records electrical events, not mechanical or contractile events.

Abnormalities
You may encounter the following variations of the P wave:
• *Peaked, biphasic, or notched and widened P waves*. These P waves may indicate atrial hypertrophy and delayed impulse conduction through the atria.
• *Inverted P waves*. Inversions in leads that are normally upright may mean that the electrical impulse is following a path outside the normal conduction system. This may lead to ectopic atrial or junctional rhythms.
• *Sawtooth-patterned P waves*. Broad, notched P waves may indicate atrial flutter.

• *Absent P waves*. Absent P waves may indicate junctional rhythms or atrial fibrillation. When a P wave doesn't precede the QRS complex, complete heart block may be present.
• *Varying P waves*. If the shapes and sizes of the P waves vary, the impulses may be originating at more than one pacemaker site within the atria.

Tp wave

The Tp (or Ta) wave represents atrial repolarization and is deflected in the direction opposite the P wave. Thus, if the P wave is upright, the Tp wave will be inverted.

Usually, you won't be able to see the Tp wave because the QRS complex obscures it.

PR interval

The PR interval represents atrial and atrioventricular (AV) conduction time. This includes atrial depolarization, the normal conduction delay in the AV node, and the passage of the electrical impulse through the bundle of His and the bundle branches. A normal PR interval will have the following characteristics:
• *Location*. Extends from the beginning of the P wave to the beginning of the Q wave in the QRS complex. If no Q wave exists, measure to the beginning of the R wave in the QRS complex.
• *Configuration*. Not applicable.
• *Amplitude*. Not applicable.
• *Duration*. 0.12 to 0.20 second.
• *Deflection*. Not applicable.

Significance
Changes in the PR interval may indicate an altered impulse formation or a conduction delay, as seen in AV block.

Abnormalities
You may encounter the following abnormalities in the duration of the PR interval:
• *Prolonged PR interval*. A prolonged PR interval may signify a conduction delay through the AV junction or a conduction delay through the

atria. A prolonged PR interval may also be a normal variation.

• *Shortened PR interval.* The PR interval may be shortened in AV junctional rhythms and pre-excitation syndromes. It's also a normal variation in infants.

QRS complex

The QRS complex represents ventricular depolarization. Although atrial repolarization usually occurs at the same time, it's not visible on the ECG. A normal QRS complex will have the following characteristics:

• *Location.* Follows the PR interval.
• *Configuration.* The QRS complex consists of three waves: the Q wave, the first negative deflection in the complex; the R wave, the positive deflection; and the S wave, the negative deflection after the R wave. Remember that not all QRS complexes will have all three waves. Because the ventricles depolarize quickly, minimizing the contact time between the stylus and ECG paper, the QRS complex typically appears thinner than other ECG components. It also typically looks different in each lead.
• *Amplitude.* 5 mm to 30 mm. When documenting specific waves in the QRS complex, use uppercase letters to indicate a wave larger than 5 mm; use lowercase letters to indicate a wave smaller than 5 mm.
• *Duration.* 0.04 to 0.10 second.
• *Deflection.* Positive in leads I, II, III, aV_L, aV_F, V_4, V_5, and V_6. Negative in leads aV_R, V_1, V_2, and V_3.

Significance
Identifying and correctly interpreting the QRS complex is crucial in assessing ventricular myocardial cell activity. The QRS complex indicates that the electrical impulse has arrived in the terminal Purkinje fibers. The impulse is then rapidly distributed to the ventricular muscle fibers, causing ventricular depolarization. Partway through the inscription of the QRS complex onto the ECG paper, the ventricles start to contract. If you watch the ECG monitor and take your patient's pulse simulta-

neously, you'll see the QRS complex first, and a fraction of a second later you'll be able to feel the patient's pulse.

Abnormalities
You may encounter any of these QRS complex variations:

• *Deep or widened Q waves.* If the Q-wave amplitude is 25% of the R-wave amplitude or the duration of the Q wave is 0.04 second or more, the patient may have a myocardial infarction (MI).
• *QRS configuration variations.* A notched R wave may indicate a bundle-branch block.
• *Widened QRS complex.* A QRS complex greater than 0.10 second indicates that conduction has been delayed in the ventricles. This may happen with bundle-branch blocks, premature ventricular contractions, and idioventricular rhythms.
• *Missing QRS complex.* If a QRS complex doesn't appear after each P wave, the patient may be experiencing ventricular standstill.

ST segment

This isoelectric segment represents the end of ventricular depolarization and the beginning of ventricular repolarization. The point marking the end of the QRS complex and the beginning of the ST segment is known as the J point. A normal ST segment will have the following characteristics:

• *Location.* Follows the QRS complex, extending from the end of the S wave to the beginning of the T wave.
• *Configuration.* Not applicable.
• *Amplitude.* Not applicable.
• *Duration.* Not measured.
• *Deflection.* Usually isoelectric, but may vary from −0.5 to +1 mm in some precordial leads. When you evaluate the ST segment, remember that its most important characteristic is its deflection. If the ST segment is more than 1 mm above the baseline, consider it elevated. If it's more than 1 mm below, consider it depressed.

Significance

A change in a patient's ST segment may indicate myocardial damage.

Abnormalities

You may encounter the following abnormalities in the ST segment:
• *Elevation.* An ST-segment elevation of 2 mm or more may indicate myocardial injury or early repolarization.
• *Depression.* An ST-segment depression may indicate myocardial injury or ischemia. It may also result from digitalis use. A concave ST segment may indicate digitalis toxicity.

T wave

The T wave represents ventricular repolarization or recovery. A normal T wave will have the following characteristics:
• *Location.* Follows the ST segment.
• *Configuration.* Slightly rounded and smooth.
• *Amplitude.* Up to 5 mm in leads I, II, and III, and up to 10 mm in the precordial leads.
• *Duration.* Not measured.
• *Deflection.* Upright in leads I, II, V_3, V_4, V_5, and V_6. Inverted in aV_R. Variable in all other leads.

Significance

The peak of the T wave represents the relative refractory period of ventricular repolarization. Bumps in a T wave may mean that a P wave is hidden in it. In this case, atrial depolarization has occurred, so the impulse has originated at a site above the ventricles.

Abnormalities

You may encounter any of the following T-wave abnormalities:
• *Notched or pointed T waves.* Heavily notched or sharply pointed T waves in adults may indicate pericarditis or an MI.
• *Tall T waves.* These T waves suggest an MI or elevated potassium levels.
• *Inverted T waves.* A negative T wave in leads I, II, V_3, V_4, V_5, or V_6 may indicate myocardial ischemia.

QT interval

A combination of the QRS complex and the ST segment, the QT interval represents ventricular depolarization and repolarization. A normal QT interval will have the following characteristics:
• *Location.* Measured from the beginning of the QRS complex to the end of the T wave.
• *Configuration.* Not applicable.
• *Amplitude.* Not applicable.
• *Duration.* Usually between 0.36 and 0.44 second, but varies greatly depending on patient's heart rate, sex, and age. The duration also fluctuates during sleep. The QT interval should be less than half the distance between consecutive R waves (called the R-R interval) when the rhythm is regular.
• *Deflection.* Not applicable.

Significance

The QT interval shows the time needed for the ventricular depolarization-repolarization cycle. An abnormal duration may indicate a myocardial problem.

Abnormalities

You may detect these abnormalities in the QT interval:
• *Prolonged QT interval.* This indicates prolonged ventricular repolarization, which means the relative refractory period is longer. A prolonged QT interval may be of congenital or familial origin. It may also result from certain medications, particularly Group I antiarrhythmics, and is commonly seen in patients with spontaneous intracranial or subarachnoid hemorrhage.
• *Shortened QT interval.* This variation may result from hypercalcemia or digitalis toxicity.

U wave

The U wave appears to represent the repolarization of the papillary muscles or the Purkinje fibers. When present, a normal U wave has the following characteristics:
• *Location.* Follows the T wave.

Determining rhythm: Two methods

Use one of the methods described below to determine your patient's atrial and ventricular rhythms.

Paper and pencil method

Place the electrocardiogram (ECG) strip on a flat surface, then position the straight edge of a piece of paper along the strip's baseline. Now, move the paper up slightly so the straight edge is near the peak of the P waves. With a pencil, make dots on the paper at the first two P waves. Next, move the paper across the strip from left to right, lining up the two dots with succeeding P waves. If the distance for each P wave is the same, the atrial rhythm is regular. If the distance varies, the rhythm is irregular.

Using the same method, measure the distance between the R waves of consecutive QRS complexes (the R-R interval) to determine whether the ventricular rhythm is regular or irregular.

Calipers method

With the ECG strip on a flat surface, place one point of the ECG calipers on the peak of the first P wave. Then, adjust the caliper legs so the other point is on the peak of the next P wave. This distance is the P-P interval. Now, move the calipers, placing the first point on the peak of the second P wave. Note whether the other point is on the peak of the third P wave. Check the succeeding P waves in this manner. If all the intervals are the same, the atrial rhythm is regular; if the intervals vary by more than 0.04 second, the rhythm is irregular.

Using the same method, measure the R-R intervals of consecutive QRS complexes to determine whether the ventricular rhythm is regular or irregular.

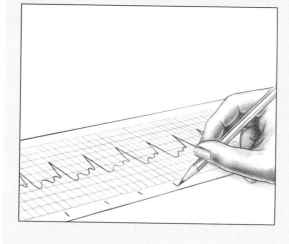

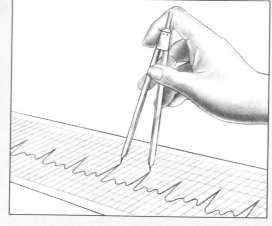

- *Configuration.* Small and rounded.
- *Amplitude.* Not measured.
- *Duration.* Not measured.
- *Deflection.* Usually upright.

Significance

The U wave may or may not appear on the ECG. When it does appear, it may be abnormal depending on its configuration.

Abnormalities

You may encounter the following U-wave abnormalities:

- *Prominent U wave.* This variation may result from hypercalcemia, potassium deficiency, digitalis toxicity, and exercise.

Analyzing ECGs

Several methods have been developed for analyzing ECGs, including the five-step method, which is described below. When you interpret an ECG, you can use this or any reliable method. Remember, the method itself isn't crucial; following it consistently is.

Five-step method

Begin the five-step method by looking over the entire rhythm strip and identifying the components of the waveform. As you look at the waveform, briefly note the configuration of each wave.

Then follow the five steps: determine the rhythm, determine the rate, evaluate conduction, evaluate other components, and interpret your findings.

Step 1: Determine the rhythm
To determine atrial and ventricular rhythms, use either the paper and pencil method or the calipers method. (See *Determining rhythm: Two methods.*) To determine the atrial rhythm, measure the intervals between consecutive P waves. These P-P intervals should occur regularly with only small variations, no more than 0.04 second. Make sure you haven't overlooked any P waves hidden in an ST segment or a T wave. Compare the P-P intervals in several cycles. If they're occurring regularly, the atrial rate is regular. Dissimilar P-P intervals indicate an irregular atrial rhythm. If the irregularity occurs in a distinct pattern, the atrial rhythm is referred to as regularly irregular. This may indicate atrial quadrigeminy.

To determine the ventricular rhythm, measure the intervals between consecutive R waves in the QRS complexes. If an R wave isn't present, use either the Q wave or the S wave of the QRS complex. The R-R intervals should occur regularly. Compare R-R intervals in several cycles. As with the atrial rhythm, similar intervals indicate a regular rhythm, dissimilar intervals indicate an irregular rhythm, and ir-

regularity occurring in a distinct pattern indicates a regularly irregular rhythm.

Step 2: Determine the rate
You can use one of two methods to determine the atrial and ventricular heart rates on an ECG. Although these methods should provide accurate information, don't rely solely on them when assessing your patient. Remember, the ECG waveform represents electrical activity— *not* mechanical activity. An ECG can show you that ventricular depolarization has taken place, but it doesn't show you that ventricular contraction has occurred. To confirm that, you must take the patient's pulse. So, always correlate the patient's heart rate as determined by the ECG with his pulse rate.

To determine the atrial rate, count the number of P waves in a 6-second rhythm strip and multiply this by 10. Probably the simplest technique, the *times ten method* proves useful if the patient's heart rhythm is irregular. Determine the ventricular rate in the same way, but count the number of QRS complexes in the same 6-second period. Multiply by 10.

You can use the second method, called the *box method,* when your patient's heart rhythm is regular. First, select identical points on two consecutive P waves. Next, count the number of small boxes between these two points. Then divide 1,500 by the number of boxes. This gives you the atrial rate per minute (because 1,500 small boxes equal 1 minute). For example, if you count 15 small boxes from the peak of one P wave to the peak of the next P wave, and divide 1,500 by 15, you'll find that the atrial rate is 100. To calculate the ventricular rate, use the same method, but with two consecutive R waves.

Step 3: Evaluate conduction
To evaluate conduction, you must measure three ECG components: the PR interval, the QRS complex, and the QT interval. In the process of measuring these components, you'll also evaluate the P wave and the T wave.

P wave and QRS complex: Noting the pattern

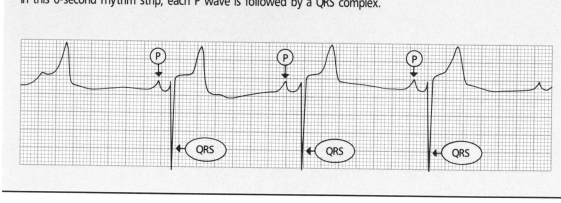

In this 6-second rhythm strip, each P wave is followed by a QRS complex.

PR interval

Before you can measure the PR interval, you must evaluate the P waves. Note whether all P waves have a normal configuration. Are they similar in size and shape? Does a QRS complex follow every P wave? (See *P wave and QRS complex: Noting the pattern.*)

If you detect a P wave for every QRS complex, examine the PR interval. If not, note how often a P wave isn't followed by a QRS complex. This could indicate Type II second-degree heart block or complete heart block.

To determine the PR interval, count the small squares between the start of the P wave and the start of the QRS complex, then multiply the number of squares by 0.04 second. Is the duration of the PR interval within normal limits—0.12 to 0.20 second (three to five small squares)? If not, is it prolonged or shortened? The PR interval will be prolonged in sinus rhythm with first-degree heart block, and it will be shortened in some junctional rhythms.

Is the PR interval constant? Be sure to measure three or four consecutive PR intervals to make sure they're the same. Describe any variations. A pattern of irregularity may indicate Type I second-degree AV heart block.

QRS complex

When measuring the QRS complex duration, always start at the end of the PR interval and measure straight across to the end of the S wave. Be sure to measure to the end of this wave, not just to its peak. And remember that a QRS complex has no horizontal components. (See *Measuring the QRS complex.*)

Count the number of small squares between the beginning and the end of the QRS complex, and multiply by 0.04 second. Then note whether the duration falls within normal limits (0.04 to 0.10 second). Are all QRS complexes the same size and shape? If not, describe each variation. Also, note whether all QRS complexes have the same duration. If not, note the duration of each.

QT interval

Before you can measure the duration of the QT interval, you must evaluate the T waves on the rhythm strip. Do all of them have a normal shape and amplitude? Do they have the same deflection as the QRS complexes?

The QT interval begins with the Q wave (or the R wave if no Q wave exists) and ends at the termination of the T wave. Count the number of small squares between the beginning of the QRS complex and the end of the T wave (where the T wave returns to the baseline). Then multiply the number of squares by

Measuring the QRS complex

Determining the duration of a QRS complex can be difficult. Here the shaded areas show you exactly where the QRS complexes begin and end.

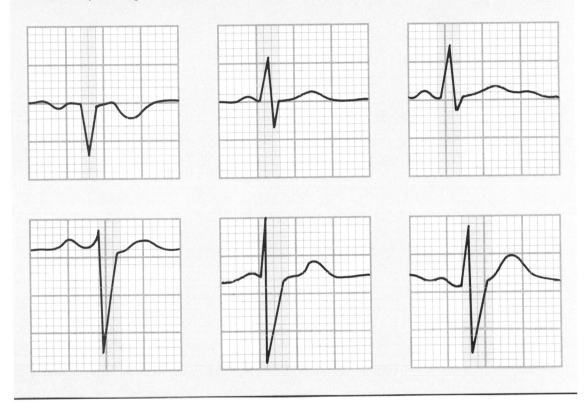

0.04 second. Note whether the QT intervals fall within normal limits—0.36 to 0.44 second.

Step 4: Evaluate other components
In this step, observe any other components on the ECG strip. Note any ectopic or aberrantly conducted beats and other abnormalities. Also, check the ST segment for any abnormalities and look for a U wave.

During this step, you should also recheck the configuration, amplitude, and duration of the P wave, the QRS complex, and the T wave.

Step 5: Interpret your findings
In this final step, describe your findings for each component of the rhythm strip. Using words—not just figures—will help you identify the rhythm that you're analyzing.

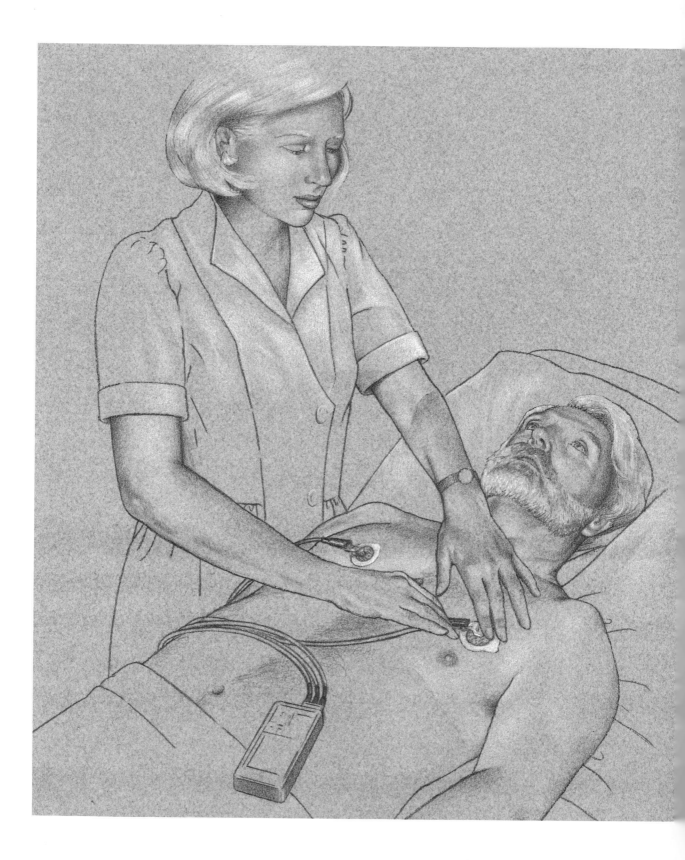

3

CHAPTER

Single-lead monitoring

Each electrocardiogram (ECG) lead gives you a distinct view of the heart's electrical activity, and a 12-lead ECG provides a broader picture of this activity. But because a 12-lead ECG can be uncomfortable for the patient, and may provide more information than you need, you'll frequently use single-lead monitoring. Typically, a 12-lead ECG is used to diagnose a cardiac condition and interpret a cardiac rhythm, whereas a single lead is used to monitor the patient's cardiac rhythm on an ongoing basis.

This chapter will focus on single-lead continuous monitoring, in which one lead, or view of the heart, is monitored at a time. Specifically, the chapter covers the two types of single-lead monitoring: hardwire and telemetry. You'll also read about which leads are most appropriate for monitoring patients with various cardiac conditions. And in the last section of the chapter, you'll find a review of how to obtain a single-lead rhythm strip.

Using a five-leadwire system

This illustration shows the correct placement of the five electrodes or leadwires. The electrodes are color coded as follows:
• white—right arm (RA)
• black—left arm (LA)
• green—right leg (RL)
• red—left leg (LL)
• brown—chest (C).
   In this illustration, the brown chest electrode is in the V_1 position. You can place this leadwire in any of the six chest lead positions.

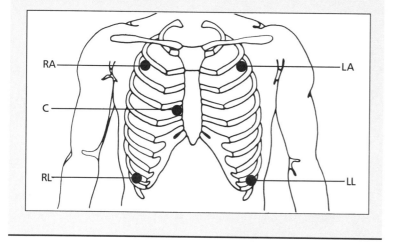

Types of monitoring

Although single-lead monitoring doesn't give you a complete picture of the heart's electrical activity, it does give you a continuous one, which can be crucial to understanding a patient's cardiac status. You can monitor a single lead using either hardwire monitoring or telemetry (wireless monitoring). The choice will depend on several factors, including whether the patient is ambulatory and the particular lead you want to monitor.

   The leads in single-lead monitoring approximate those in 12-lead monitoring. But the electrode positions for the limb leads differ. With single-lead monitoring, you place the limb lead electrodes on the chest.

Hardwire monitoring

You may perform hardwire monitoring using one of several systems available. The most common hardwire monitoring systems are the five-leadwire system and the three-leadwire system.

Five-leadwire system

With the five-leadwire system, you can monitor your patient in any of the standard 12 leads. This includes the leads requiring two electrodes (called bipolar leads)—leads I, II, and III—and leads requiring only one electrode (called unipolar leads)—leads aV_R, aV_L, aV_F, V_1, V_2, V_3, V_4, V_5, and V_6. Besides these standard leads, you can also monitor the modified chest leads MCL_1 and MCL_6, which simulate leads V_1 and V_6. These modified leads are bipolar. Two other leads, the Lewis lead and the sternal lead, may also be viewed with a five-leadwire system.

   To use the five-leadwire system, place the color-coded electrodes in the following areas:
• white electrode—below the right clavicle
• black electrode—below the left clavicle
• green electrode—on the right lower anterior rib cage
• red electrode—on the left lower anterior rib cage
• brown electrode—in one of the chest (or precordial) lead positions (V_1 through V_6).
   The six chest lead positions include:
• V_1—fourth intercostal space at the right sternal border
• V_2—fourth intercostal space at the left sternal border
• V_3—midway between V_2 and V_4
• V_4—fifth intercostal space at the left midclavicular line
• V_5—fifth intercostal space at the left anterior axillary line
• V_6—fifth intercostal space at the left midaxillary line.
(See *Using a five-leadwire system*.)
   With the electrodes in place, you can monitor the limb leads simply by changing the lead selector on the machine. To monitor a chest lead, you must place the brown electrode in

the appropriate position and change the lead selector.

Three-leadwire system

With the three-leadwire system, you can monitor the bipolar leads I, II, and III. To do so, place the color-coded electrodes in the following areas:
• white electrode—below the right clavicle
• black electrode—below the left clavicle
• red electrode—on the left lower anterior rib cage.

After you've placed the electrodes, simply turn the lead selector to the appropriate setting for lead I, II, or III. (See *Using a three-leadwire system.*)

Although you can't monitor the chest leads with a three-leadwire system, you can monitor the bipolar modified chest leads, which provide similar information. To monitor any of these leads, turn the lead selector switch to lead III. Then reposition the red electrode to the appropriate position for the chest lead you want to monitor. For example, to monitor MCL_1, you'd turn the lead selector switch to lead III. Then you'd move the red electrode to the fourth intercostal space at the right sternal border (the V_1 position).

Telemetry

Wireless monitoring, or telemetry, gives your patient more freedom than the 12-lead system or the hardwire monitoring system. With telemetry, you attach two or three electrodes to your patient's chest. But instead of being connected to a bedside monitor, the patient carries a small transmitter. With some telemetry equipment, the ECG waveforms will be labeled on the screen at a central monitoring station.

With telemetry, you'll have one positive electrode, one negative electrode and, possibly, a ground electrode. Most commonly, you'll monitor either lead MCL_1 or lead II. To monitor lead MCL_1, place the electrodes as follows:
• negative electrode—below the left clavicle
• positive electrode—fourth intercostal space at the right sternal border
• ground electrode—below the right clavicle.

Using a three-leadwire system

This illustration shows you where to place the electrodes to monitor leads I, II, and III, using a three-leadwire system. The electrodes are color coded as follows:
• white—right arm (RA)
• black—left arm (LA)
• red—left leg (LL).

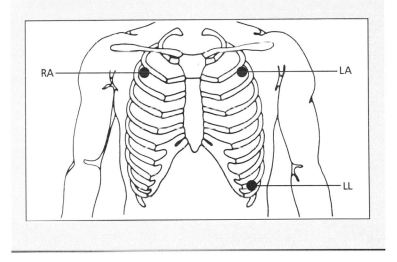

To monitor lead II, place the electrodes as follows:
• negative electrode—below the right clavicle
• positive electrode—left lower anterior rib cage
• ground electrode—below the left clavicle.

Selecting a lead

The lead you choose to monitor will vary depending on several factors. Chief among them will be the patient's particular cardiac problem and the capabilities of the monitoring systems available to you. In this section, you'll find the leads you're most likely to use along with brief descriptions of the ECG characteristics and the patient conditions they best detect. (See *Creating monitoring leads,* pages 34 and 35.)

(Text continues on page 36.)

Creating monitoring leads

This chart shows the correct electrode positions for some of the monitoring leads you'll use most often. For each lead, you'll see electrode placement for a five-leadwire system, a three-leadwire system, and a telemetry system.

In the two hardwire systems, the electrode positions for one lead may be identical to the electrode positions for another lead. In this case, you simply change the lead selector switch to the set-ting that corresponds to the lead you want. In some cases, you'll need to reposition the electrodes.

In the telemetry system, you can create the same lead with two electrodes that you do with three, simply by eliminating the ground electrode.

The chart uses these abbreviations: RA, right arm; LA, left arm; RL, right leg; LL, left leg; C, chest; and G, ground.

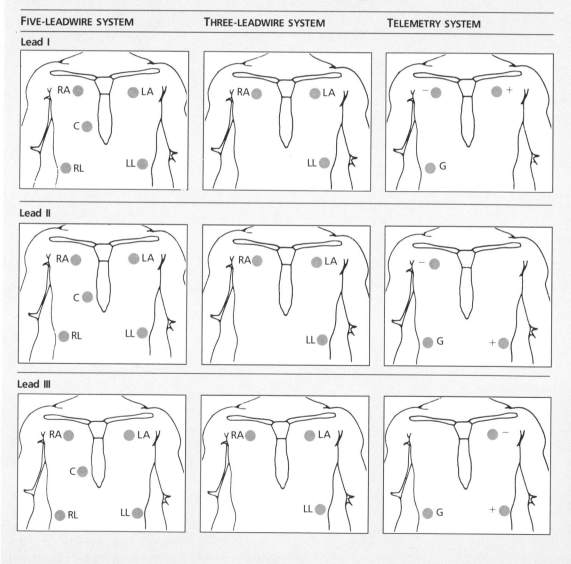

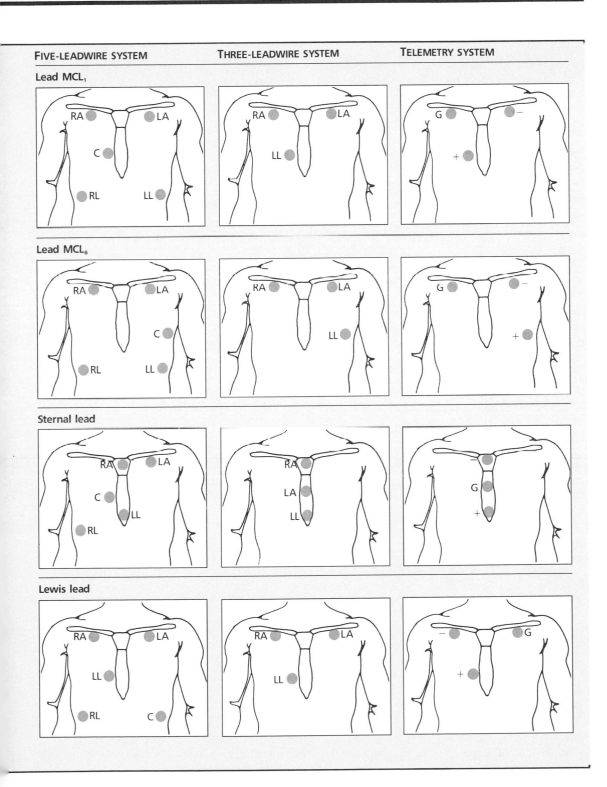

FIVE-LEADWIRE SYSTEM   THREE-LEADWIRE SYSTEM   TELEMETRY SYSTEM

Lead MCL$_1$

Lead MCL$_6$

Sternal lead

Lewis lead

Using simultaneous dual monitoring

Monitoring in two leads provides a more complete picture than monitoring in one. With simultaneous dual monitoring, you'll generally review the first lead—usually designated as the primary lead—for arrhythmias. A two-lead view also helps detect episodic ectopic beats or rhythms. Leads II and V_1 are the two leads most often monitored simultaneously.

Lead II

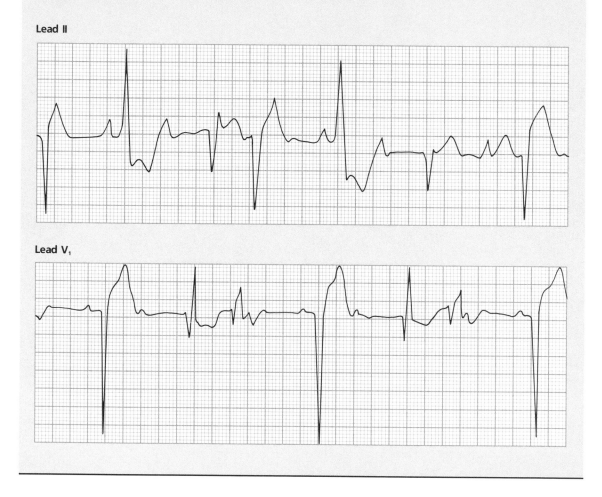

Lead V_1

Lead MCL$_1$
A bipolar lead, MCL$_1$ is one of the more commonly monitored leads. You'll use it when you want to focus on the P wave. You'll also select lead MCL$_1$ when you're monitoring one of the following problems:
• supraventricular impulses
• atrial hypertrophy
• bundle-branch block
• ventricular ectopy.

Lead MCL$_1$ can help in distinguishing right and left bundle-branch block as well as right and left ventricular ectopy. One key disadvantage of lead MCL$_1$ is that it can't detect shifts in the axis.

Sometimes, you may monitor lead MCL$_1$ as part of a technique known as simultaneous dual monitoring. (See *Using simultaneous dual monitoring*.)

Leads MCL$_2$ through MCL$_6$
These bipolar simulations of unipolar leads V$_2$ through V$_6$ are your best choices when you're monitoring a patient with a myocardial injury or infarction. They're especially useful when the anterior or lateral left ventricle wall is affected.

Lead V$_1$
You can monitor this unipolar lead only with a five-leadwire system. Lead V$_1$ shows the P wave, the QRS complex, and the ST segment particularly well. You may choose this lead when you're monitoring a patient with one of the following:
• ventricular arrhythmias
• ST-segment changes
• bundle-branch block
• ventricular ectopy.

This lead helps in distinguishing between right and left ventricular ectopy.

Leads V$_2$ and V$_3$
To monitor these two chest leads, you need a five-leadwire system. You can use these leads to detect ST-segment elevation, which is associated with anterior wall ischemia.

Leads V$_4$ and V$_5$
You may select one of these chest leads to monitor either ST-segment abnormalities or T-wave abnormalities.

Lead I
You'll find this unipolar limb lead particularly helpful when you're monitoring atrial rhythms and hemiblocks.

Lead II
One of the most frequently used leads, lead II will help you see large, upright P, R, and T waves.

Lewis lead
You can view this lead with either of the hardwire methods or with telemetry. The Lewis lead can help you detect the varying P waves that are associated with atrial arrhythmias.

Sternal lead
This lead is particularly useful in telemetry monitoring because it stabilizes the ECG pattern even when the patient is active. Such stabilization results from electrode placement directly on the sternum, which hardly moves during activity.

Obtaining a rhythm strip

When you need to obtain a single-lead rhythm strip, remember that careful preparation helps ensure reliable results. So be sure to prepare the patient and apply the electrodes correctly before you run a rhythm strip. After you obtain the strip, note whether you're experiencing monitor problems, such as electrical interference. If so, take the appropriate steps to correct the problems.

Preparing the patient
Turn on the bedside monitor, and as it warms up, talk to your patient. Reducing his anxiety will help ensure accurate results. Explain the monitoring procedure, and answer any questions he has. Sometimes patients think that the purpose of ECG monitoring is to control their heart rhythm. Make sure your patient understands that you're monitoring, not controlling, his heart's electrical activity. Tell him that if he hears an alarm during the procedure, it may mean that a leadwire has come loose.

Applying the electrodes
Next, prepare the patient's skin at the electrode sites. Remember, inadequately prepared skin can hamper conduction. Clean the skin with soap and water or 70% isopropyl alcohol to remove skin oil. Then allow the skin to dry thoroughly. If necessary, shave or clip the hair around the site. If the patient is perspiring, apply a commercial antiperspirant spray or tincture of benzoin.

Next, open the electrode disk packets. If a disk is no longer moist with conductive gel, discard the electrode. Apply the disks to the

Identifying cardiac monitor problems

PROBLEM	POSSIBLE CAUSES	NURSING INTERVENTIONS
Artifact (waveform interference)	• Patient experiencing seizures, chills, or anxiety	• If the patient is having a seizure, notify the doctor and intervene as ordered.
	• Patient restless	• Keep the patient warm and encourage him to relax.
	• Dirty or corroded connections	• Replace dirty or corroded wires.
	• Improper electrode application	• Check the electrodes and reapply them if needed. Clean the patient's skin well because skin oils and dead skin cells inhibit conduction.
		• Check the electrode gel. If the gel is dry, apply new electrodes.
	• Electrical short circuit in leadwires or cable	• Replace broken equipment.
	• Electrical interference from other electrical equipment in the room	• Make sure all electrical equipment is attached to a common ground. Check all three-pronged plugs to ensure that none of the prongs is loose. Notify biomedical department.
	• Static electricity interference from inadequate room humidity	• Regulate room humidity to 40%, if possible.
False-high-rate alarm	• Gain setting too high, particularly with MCL, setting	• Assess the patient for signs and symptoms of hyperkalemia.
		• Reset gain.
		• Try repositioning the electrodes.
Weak signals	• Improper electrode application	• Reapply the electrodes.
	• QRS complex too small to register	• Reset GAIN so that the height of the complex is greater than 1 millivolt.
		• Try monitoring the patient on another lead.
	• HIGH alarm set too low, or LOW alarm set too high	• Set alarm limits according to the patient's heart rate.
	• Wire or cable failure	• Replace any faulty wires or cables.
Wandering baseline	• Patient restless	• Encourage the patient to relax.
	• Chest wall movement during respiration	• Make sure that tension on the cable isn't pulling the electrode away from the patient's body.
	• Improper electrode application; electrode positioned over bone	• Reposition improperly placed electrodes.

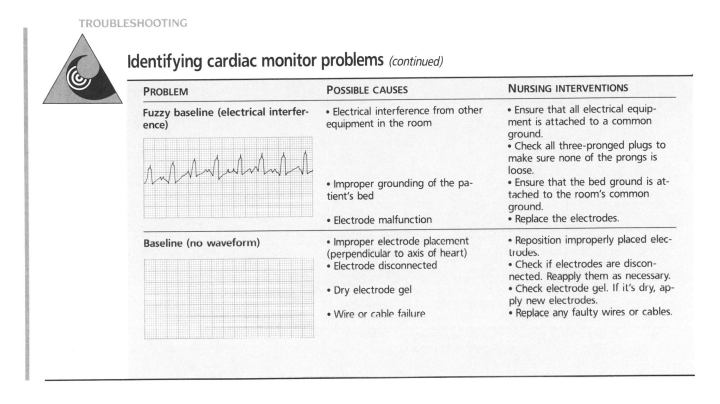

Identifying cardiac monitor problems *(continued)*

PROBLEM	POSSIBLE CAUSES	NURSING INTERVENTIONS
Fuzzy baseline (electrical interference)	• Electrical interference from other equipment in the room	• Ensure that all electrical equipment is attached to a common ground. • Check all three-pronged plugs to make sure none of the prongs is loose.
	• Improper grounding of the patient's bed	• Ensure that the bed ground is attached to the room's common ground.
	• Electrode malfunction	• Replace the electrodes.
Baseline (no waveform)	• Improper electrode placement (perpendicular to axis of heart) • Electrode disconnected	• Reposition improperly placed electrodes. • Check if electrodes are disconnected. Reapply them as necessary.
	• Dry electrode gel	• Check electrode gel. If it's dry, apply new electrodes.
	• Wire or cable failure	• Replace any faulty wires or cables.

appropriate sites, ensuring that the gel makes good contact with the skin and that the adhesive forms a tight seal. Avoid placing electrodes over bony areas, skin folds, scar tissue, and breast tissue. Insert the electrode cables into the proper receptacles in the monitor cable.

Two cautions: Make sure all the electrodes on the patient are the same brand. And change all electrodes at the same time of day—every 24 to 48 hours, as needed.

Running a rhythm strip

Now, run a rhythm strip and examine it. Your monitoring system may print nothing at the top, or it may print information such as the patient's bed number, the date and time, and the patient's heart rate.

If the ECG pattern is unreadable, you may have selected an incorrect gain size. (See *Identifying cardiac monitor problems.*) The waves, complexes, and intervals should be complete and of adequate size. If the baseline of the tracing moves up and down, make sure the electrodes are secure. Also make sure your patient is relaxed and reasonably still. If you de-

tect electrical interference, check the grounding of both the patient and the equipment. Weak signals may indicate a problem with the high or low alarm settings. These signals may also indicate faulty wiring or incorrectly placed electrodes.

If you can't determine the cardiac rhythm in one lead, switch to another. If possible, you should have 12-lead ECG equipment available, too, in case you need a complete picture of the patient's cardiac electrical activity.

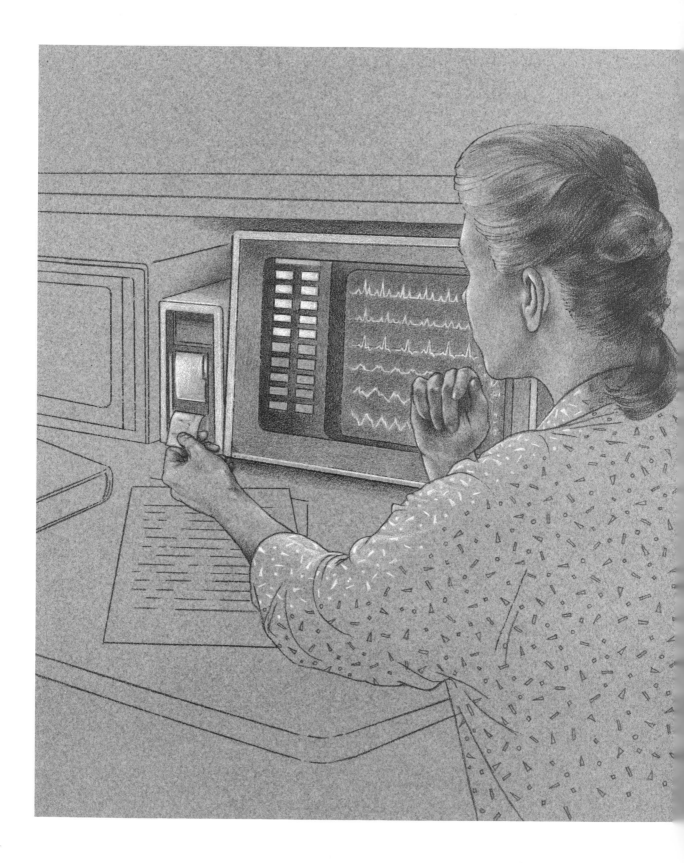

Arrhythmia recognition

Today, with cardiac monitors becoming more and more commonplace in many clinical areas, you need to know how to identify and interpret rhythm disturbances accurately — and how to intervene appropriately. This chapter, which focuses on major arrhythmias, gives you the facts you need to do both. It provides rhythm strips with distinguishing electrocardiogram (ECG) characteristics that help you identify common arrhythmias. Plus, the chapter covers causes, assessment findings, and interventions for each arrhythmia.

Types of arrhythmias

Based on the location of the electrical disturbance, arrhythmias can be classified as sinus, atrial, junctional, and ventricular arrhythmias and atrioventricular (AV) blocks.

Normally, the sinoatrial (SA) node acts as the heart's primary pacemaker, initiating the

Normal sinus rhythm

Lead II

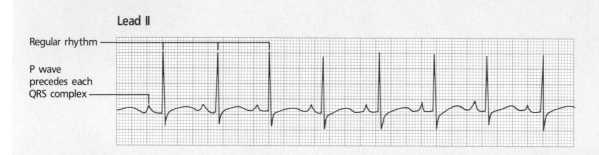

Regular rhythm

P wave
precedes each
QRS complex

Characteristics and interpretation
Atrial rhythm: regular
Ventricular rhythm: regular
Atrial rate: 60 to 100 beats/minute. On this strip, it's 80 beats/minute.
Ventricular rate: 60 to 100 beats/minute. On this strip, it's 80 beats/minute.
P wave: normally shaped. All P waves are similar in size and shape. A P wave precedes every QRS complex.
PR interval: within normal limits (0.12 to 0.20 second) and constant. On this strip, the duration is 0.20 second.
QRS complex: within normal limits (0.06 to 0.10 second). All QRS complexes have the same configuration. On this strip, the duration is 0.12 second.
T wave: normally shaped (upright and rounded). Each QRS complex is followed by a T wave.
QT interval: within normal limits (0.36 to 0.44 second) and constant. On this strip, the duration is 0.44 second.

electrical impulses that set the rhythm for cardiac contractions. The SA node assumes this role because its automatic firing rate exceeds that of the heart's other pacemakers, allowing the cells to depolarize spontaneously. Two factors account for this increased automaticity: First, during the resting phase of the depolarization-repolarization cycle, sinus node cells have the least negative charge. Second, depolarization actually begins during the resting phase. (See *Normal sinus rhythm.*)

Changes in one or both of these characteristics may lead to functional disturbances in the SA node, producing *sinus arrhythmias*. These include sinus arrhythmia, sinus bradycardia, sinus tachycardia, and sinus arrest.

Enhanced automaticity of atrial tissue or reentry may produce *atrial arrhythmias*. The most common cardiac arrhythmias, atrial arrhythmias may shorten diastole, reducing ventricular filling and coronary artery perfusion. They also may diminish atrial kick. When caused by enhanced automaticity, they may stem from digitalis toxicity, elevated catecholamine levels, hypoxia, and electrolyte abnormalities. When reentry triggers atrial arrhythmias, causes may include ischemia, electrolyte abnormalities, and use of certain drugs that result in slow, one-way impulse conduction through atrial tissue.

Junctional arrhythmias originate in the AV junction, which includes the area around the AV node and the bundle of His. These arrhythmias usually occur when a higher pacemaker is suppressed or when impulses are blocked at the AV node.

Ventricular arrhythmias originate in ventricular tissue below the bifurcation of the bundle of His. These rhythms may result from reentry, enhanced automaticity, or afterdepolarization.

An *AV block* results from an abnormal interruption or delay of atrial impulse conduction to the ventricles. It may be partial or total and may occur in the AV node, the bundle of His, or the Purkinje system. Studies have demonstrated AV block in normal hearts when atrial rates reach the range of 125 to 150 beats/minute.

Sinus arrhythmia

In sinus arrhythmia, the heart rate stays within normal limits, but the rhythm is irregular and corresponds to the respiratory cycle and variations of vagal tone. During inspiration, an increased volume of blood returns to the heart, reducing vagal tone and increasing the sinus rate. During expiration, venous return decreases, vagal tone increases, and the sinus rate slows.

Conditions unrelated to respiration may also produce sinus arrhythmia. These conditions include an inferior wall myocardial infarction (MI), digitalis toxicity, and increased intracranial pressure (ICP).

Assessment findings

Sinus arrhythmia is easily recognized in elderly, pediatric, and sedated patients. The patient's pulse rate increases with inspiration and decreases with expiration. Usually, the patient will be asymptomatic.

Intervention

Treatment usually isn't necessary, unless the patient is symptomatic or the sinus arrhythmia stems from an underlying cause. When the patient is symptomatic, atropine may be administered if the heart rate falls below 40 beats/minute.

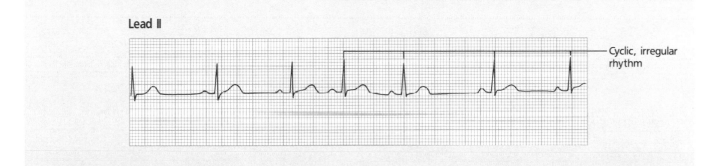

Lead II

Cyclic, irregular rhythm

Characteristics and interpretation
Atrial rhythm: irregular, corresponding to the respiratory cycle
Ventricular rhythm: irregular, corresponding to the respiratory cycle
Atrial rate: within normal limits, varies with respiration. On this strip, it's 60 beats/minute.

Ventricular rate: within normal limits, varies with respiration. On this strip, it's 60 beats/minute.
P wave: normal size and configuration. A P wave precedes each QRS complex.
PR interval: within normal limits. On this strip, it's 0.16 second and constant.
QRS complex: normal duration and

configuration. On this strip, the duration is 0.06 second.
T wave: normal size and configuration
QT interval: within normal limits. On this strip, it's 0.36 second.
Other: phasic slowing and quickening of the rhythm

Sinus bradycardia

Characterized by a sinus rate of less than 60 beats/minute, sinus bradycardia usually occurs as the normal response to a reduced demand for blood flow. It's common among athletes, whose well-conditioned hearts can maintain stroke volume with reduced effort. It may also be caused by drugs, such as digitalis, calcium channel blockers, and beta blockers.

Sinus bradycardia may occur after an inferior wall MI involving the right coronary artery, which provides the blood supply to the SA node. The rhythm may develop during sleep and in patients with elevated ICP. It may also result from vagal stimulation caused by vomiting or defecating. Pathologic sinus bradycardia may occur with sick sinus syndrome.

Assessment findings
The patient will be asymptomatic if he's able to compensate for the drop in heart rate by increasing stroke volume. If not, he may have signs and symptoms of decreased cardiac output, such as hypotension, syncope, confusion, and blurred vision.

Intervention
If the patient is asymptomatic, treatment isn't necessary. If he has signs and symptoms, treatment aims to identify and correct the underlying cause. The heart rate may be increased with such drugs as atropine or isoproterenol. A temporary or permanent pacemaker may be inserted if the bradycardia persists.

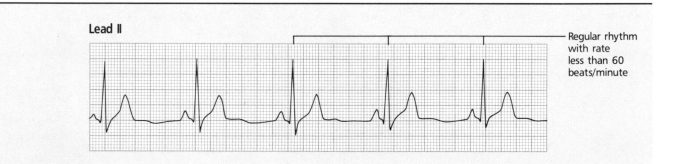

Lead II

Regular rhythm with rate less than 60 beats/minute

Characteristics and interpretation
Atrial rhythm: regular
Ventricular rhythm: regular
Atrial rate: less than 60 beats/minute. On this strip, it's 50 beats/minute.
Ventricular rate: less than 60 beats/minute. On this strip, it's 50 beats/minute.
P wave: normal size and configuration. A P wave precedes each QRS complex.
PR interval: within normal limits and constant. On this strip, the duration is 0.14 second.
QRS complex: normal duration and configuration. On this strip, the duration is 0.08 second.
T wave: normal size and configuration
QT interval: within normal limits. On this strip, it's 0.40 second.

Sinus tachycardia

A normal response to cellular demands for increased oxygen delivery and blood flow commonly produces sinus tachycardia. Conditions causing such a demand include congestive heart failure (CHF), shock, anemia, exercise, fever, hypoxia, pain, and stress. Drugs that stimulate the beta$_1$ receptors in the heart will also cause sinus tachycardia. These include isoproterenol, aminophylline, and inotropic agents, such as dopamine, dobutamine, and epinephrine. Alcohol, caffeine, and nicotine may also produce sinus tachycardia.

Sinus tachycardia, which always results from a primary problem, may be serious. An elevated heart rate increases myocardial oxygen requirements. If the patient can't meet these demands (for example, because of coronary artery disease [CAD]), ischemia and further myocardial damage may occur.

Assessment findings
The patient may complain of palpitations. Usually, however, he'll be asymptomatic.

If tachycardia persists at a rate greater than 140 beats/minute for longer than 30 minutes, you may see ST-segment and T-wave changes, indicating ischemia.

Intervention
Treatment focuses on finding the primary cause of sinus tachycardia. If the patient has high circulating catecholamine levels, a beta blocker (such as esmolol or labetalol) may be used to slow the heart rate. If the patient is recovering from an MI, persistent sinus tachycardia may warn of impending CHF or cardiogenic shock.

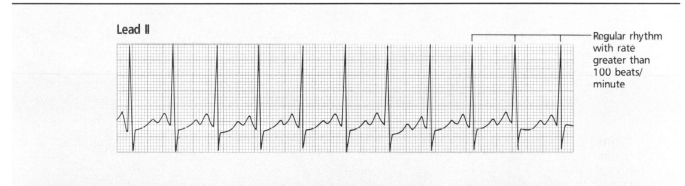

Lead II

Regular rhythm with rate greater than 100 beats/minute

Characteristics and interpretation
Atrial rhythm: regular
Ventricular rhythm: regular
Atrial rate: 100 to 160 beats/minute. On this strip, it's 110 beats/minute.
Ventricular rate: 100 to 160 beats/minute. On this strip, it's 110 beats/minute.
P wave: normal size and configuration. A P wave precedes each QRS complex. As the sinus rate reaches about 150 beats/minute, the P wave merges with the preceding T wave and may be difficult to identify. Examine the descending slope of the preceding T wave closely for notches, indicating the presence of the P wave. On this strip, the P wave is normal.
PR interval: within normal limits and constant. On this strip, the duration is 0.16 second.
QRS complex: normal duration and configuration. On this strip, the duration is 0.10 second.
T wave: normal size and configuration
QT interval: within normal limits and constant. On this strip, the duration is 0.36 second.
Other: gradual onset and cessation

Sinus arrest

Failure of the SA node to generate an impulse interrupts the sinus rhythm, producing "sinus pause" when one or two beats are dropped, or "sinus arrest" when three or more beats are dropped. Such failure may result from an acute inferior wall MI; increased vagal tone (due to increased carotid sinus sensitivity, vomiting, carotid sinus massage, or Valsalva's maneuver); or the use of certain drugs (digitalis, calcium channel blockers, or beta blockers). This arrhythmia may also be associated with sick sinus syndrome.

Assessment findings
The patient will have an irregular pulse rate associated with the sinus rhythm pauses. If the pauses are infrequent, the patient will be asymptomatic. If the pauses occur frequently and last for several seconds, the patient may have signs and symptoms of decreased cardiac output, including hypotension, confusion, syncope, and blurred vision.

Intervention
An asymptomatic patient needs no treatment. For a symptomatic patient, treatment focuses on maintaining cardiac output and discovering the cause of the sinus arrest. If indicated, atropine may be administered or a temporary or permanent pacemaker may be inserted.

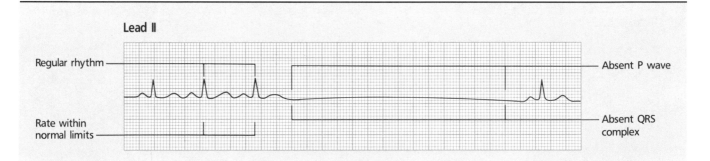

Lead II

Regular rhythm

Rate within normal limits

Absent P wave

Absent QRS complex

Characteristics and interpretation
Atrial rhythm: regular, except for the missing complex
Ventricular rhythm: regular, except for the missing complex
Atrial rate: within normal limits, but varies because of the pauses. On this strip, it's 94 beats/minute.
Ventricular rate: within normal limits, but varies because of the pauses. On this strip, it's 94 beats/minute.
P wave: normal size and configuration. A P wave precedes each QRS complex but is absent during a pause.
PR interval: within normal limits and constant when P wave is present; unmeasurable when P wave is absent. On this strip, the duration is 0.20 second on all complexes surrounding the arrest.

QRS complex: normal duration and configuration. QRS complex absent during a pause. On this strip, the duration is 0.08 second.
T wave: normal size and configuration. A T wave is absent during a pause.
QT interval: within normal limits; not measurable during a pause. On this strip, it's 0.40 second and constant.

Premature atrial contractions

Premature atrial contractions (PACs) usually result from an irritable focus in the atria that supersedes the SA node as the pacemaker for one or two beats. Although PACs commonly occur in normal hearts, they're also associated with coronary and valvular heart disease. In an inferior wall MI, PACs may indicate a concomitant right atrial infarct. In an anterior wall MI, PACs are an early sign of left ventricular failure. They also may warn of a more severe atrial arrhythmia, such as atrial flutter or fibrillation.

Possible causes include digitalis toxicity, hyperthyroidism, elevated catecholamine levels, acute respiratory failure, and chronic obstructive pulmonary disease.

Assessment findings
The patient will have an irregular pulse rate when the PACs occur. He also may complain of occasional palpitations. A patient with an anterior wall MI who displays PACs may have other signs and symptoms of diminished cardiac output, such as hypotension or syncope.

Intervention
Symptomatic patients may be treated with drugs that prolong the atrial refractory period. Such drugs include digitalis, procainamide, propranolol, and verapamil.

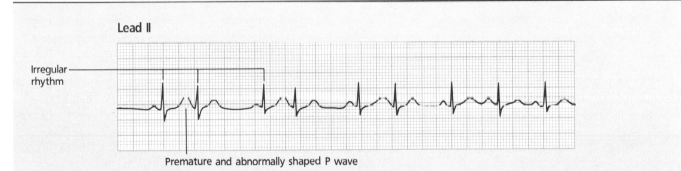

Lead II

Irregular rhythm

Premature and abnormally shaped P wave

Characteristics and interpretation
Atrial rhythm: irregular. Incomplete compensatory pause follows PAC. Underlying rhythm may be regular.
Ventricular rhythm: irregular. Incomplete compensatory pause follows PAC. Underlying rhythm may be regular.
Atrial rate: varies with underlying rhythm. On this strip, it's 90 beats/minute.
Ventricular rate: varies with underlying rhythm. On this strip, it's 90 beats/minute.
P wave: premature and abnormally shaped; possibly lost in previous T wave. Varying configurations indicate multiform PACs.
PR interval: usually within normal limits, but may be shortened or slightly prolonged, depending on the origin of the ectopic focus. On this strip, the PR interval is 0.16 second and constant.

QRS complex: usually normal duration and configuration. On this strip, it's 0.08 second and constant.
T wave: usually normal configuration; may be distorted if P wave is hidden in previous T wave.
QT interval: usually within normal limits. On this strip, it's 0.36 second and constant.
Other: may occur in bigeminy or in couplets.

Atrial tachycardia

In atrial tachycardia, the atrial rhythm is ectopic, and the atrial rate is rapid, shortening diastole. This results in a loss of atrial kick, reduced cardiac output, reduced coronary perfusion, and ischemic myocardial changes.

Although atrial tachycardia does occur in patients with normal hearts, it's usually associated with primary or secondary cardiac problems. These include high catecholamine levels, digitalis toxicity, MI, cardiomyopathy, hyperthyroidism, systemic hypertension, and valvular heart disease. This rhythm also may be a component of sick sinus syndrome.

Three types of atrial tachycardia exist: atrial tachycardia with block; multifocal atrial tachycardia (or chaotic atrial rhythm); and paroxysmal atrial tachycardia. (See *Identifying types of atrial tachycardia.*)

Assessment findings

The patient may complain of palpitations, shortness of breath, and chest pain. Decreased cardiac output may produce syncope, blurred vision, and hypotension.

Intervention

If immediate therapy is needed, the doctor may order measures to produce vagal stimulation, such as carotid sinus massage, Valsalva's maneuver, or baroreceptor reflex stimulation.

Drug therapy may include administering adenosine to stop atrial tachycardia; verapamil, digitalis, beta blockers, or edrophonium to increase the AV block; and quinidine or procainamide to establish a normal sinus rhythm.

When other treatments fail, cardioversion may be used to stop the arrhythmia. Following open-heart surgery, atrial overdrive pacing (also called burst pacing) is often necessary.

Lead II

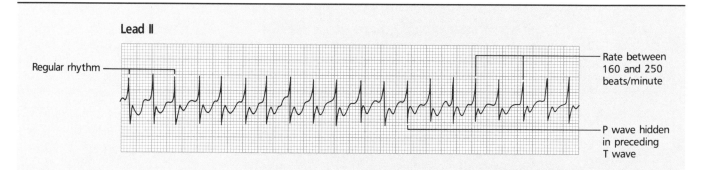

Regular rhythm

Rate between 160 and 250 beats/minute

P wave hidden in preceding T wave

Characteristics and interpretation
Atrial rhythm: regular
Ventricular rhythm: regular
Atrial rate: three or more successive ectopic atrial beats at a rate of 160 to 250 beats/minute. On this strip, it's 210 beats/minute.
Ventricular rate: varies with AV conduction ratio. On this strip, it's 210 beats/minute.
P wave: 1:1 ratio with QRS complex, though frequently not discernible due to rapid rate. May be hidden in previous ST segment or T wave.
PR interval: may be unmeasurable if P wave can't be distinguished from preceding T wave. If P wave is present, PR interval is often greater than 0.20 second due to rapid rate and intrinsic refractoriness of the AV node. On this strip, PR interval is not discernible.
QRS complex: usually normal unless aberrant intraventricular conduction is present. On this strip, the duration is 0.10 second.
T wave: may be normal or inverted if ischemia is present. On this strip, the T waves are inverted.
QT interval: usually within normal limits, but may be shorter due to rapid rate. On this strip, it's 0.20 second.
Other: ST-segment and T-wave changes appear if tachyarrhythmia persists longer than 30 minutes, indicating myocardial ischemia.

Identifying types of atrial tachycardia

These rhythm strips show you how to recognize three types of atrial tachycardia.

Atrial tachycardia with block
Increased automaticity of atrial tissue causes this arrhythmia. As the atrial rate speeds up and AV conduction becomes impaired, Type I (Mobitz I or Wenckebach) second-degree AV block may follow.

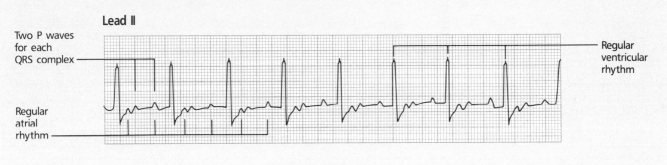

Lead II

Two P waves for each QRS complex —

Regular atrial rhythm —

— Regular ventricular rhythm

Multifocal atrial tachycardia
In this arrhythmia, atrial tachycardia occurs with multiple atrial foci. Usually, you'll see multifocal atrial tachycardia in patients with chronic pulmonary disease.

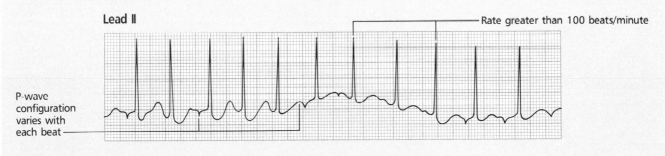

Lead II

— Rate greater than 100 beats/minute

P-wave configuration varies with each beat —

Paroxysmal atrial tachycardia
In this arrhythmia, brief periods of tachycardia alternate with periods of normal sinus rhythm. It starts and stops suddenly, with the sudden onset resulting from rapid firing of an ectopic focus.

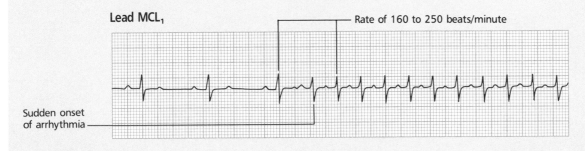

Lead MCL₁

— Rate of 160 to 250 beats/minute

Sudden onset of arrhythmia —

Atrial flutter

Characterized by an atrial rate of 300 or more beats/minute, atrial flutter results from multiple reentry circuits within the atrial tissue. Causes include conditions that enlarge atrial tissue and elevate atrial pressures. Atrial flutter is associated with MI, increased catecholamine levels, hyperthyroidism, and digitalis toxicity.

A ventricular response rate of 300 beats/minute suggests the presence of an anomalous pathway.

Assessment findings
If the patient's pulse rate is normal, he usually has no symptoms. If his pulse rate is high, he'll probably have signs and symptoms of de-creased cardiac output, such as hypotension and syncope.

Intervention
The doctor may perform vagal stimulation to slow the ventricular response and demonstrate the presence of flutter waves. Cardioversion remains the treatment of choice.

Unless an anomalous pathway is suspected, drug therapy may include verapamil or digitalis to slow the ventricular rate. If atrial flutter results from digitalis toxicity, of course, that drug wouldn't be used. After digitalization, procainamide or quinidine may also be given to establish a normal rhythm.

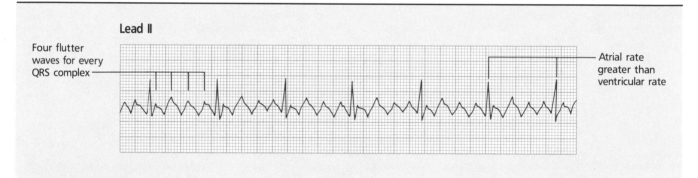

Lead II

Four flutter waves for every QRS complex

Atrial rate greater than ventricular rate

Characteristics and interpretation
Atrial rhythm: regular
Ventricular rhythm: may be regular or irregular, depending on the conduction ratio. On this strip, it's regular.
Atrial rate: 300 to 350 beats/minute. On this strip, it's 300 beats/minute.

Ventricular rate: variable. On this strip, it's 70 beats/minute.
P wave: atrial activity seen as flutter waves, often with a saw-toothed appearance
PR interval: not measurable

QRS complex: usually normal, but can be distorted by the underlying flutter waves. On this strip, the duration is 0.10 second and normal.
T wave: not identifiable
QT interval: can't be measured

Atrial fibrillation

Defined as chaotic, asynchronous, electrical activity in the atrial tissue, atrial fibrillation results from impulses in many reentry pathways. These impulses cause the atria to quiver instead of contract regularly. With this arrhythmia, blood may pool in the left atrial appendage and form thrombi that can be ejected into the systemic circulation. An associated rapid ventricular rate can decrease cardiac output.

Possible causes include valvular disorders, hypertension, CAD, MI, and the use of certain drugs, such as aminophylline and digitalis.

Assessment findings
The patient will have an irregular pulse rhythm with a normal or abnormal rate. If the ventricular rate is over 90 beats/minute, the patient will probably have a pulse deficit. The patient also may have signs and symptoms of decreased cardiac output (hypotension, syncope) and cerebral or peripheral emboli.

Intervention
Treatment aims to slow the ventricular response and improve cardiac output. If the patient is symptomatic, synchronized cardioversion should be used immediately. Vagal stimulation may be used to slow the ventricular response, but it won't convert the arrhythmia.

Certain drugs—such as diltiazem, verapamil, and digitalis—may be given to slow conduction through the AV node. Other antiarrhythmic drugs may be used to restore the sinus rhythm once the ventricular response has been slowed.

Unless contraindicated, the patient should receive anticoagulant therapy to prevent a cerebrovascular accident. He should also have regular neurologic assessments.

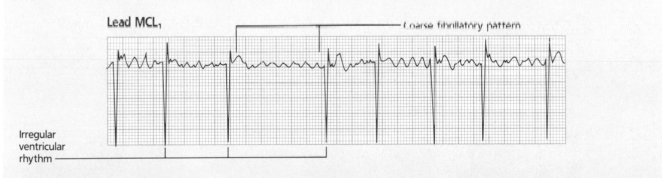

Lead MCL₁

Coarse fibrillatory pattern

Irregular ventricular rhythm

Characteristics and interpretation
Atrial rhythm: grossly irregular
Ventricular rhythm: grossly irregular
Atrial rate: greater than 400 beats/minute
Ventricular rate: 60 to 150 beats/minute, depending on treatment regimen. On this strip, it's 80 beats/minute.

P wave: absent; erratic baseline f waves (fibrillatory waves) appear in their place. When the f waves are pronounced, the arrhythmia is called coarse atrial fibrillation. When the f waves aren't pronounced, the arrhythmia is known as fine atrial fibrillation. On this strip, the f waves are pronounced.

PR interval: indiscernible
QRS complex: duration usually within normal limits, with aberrant intraventricular conduction. On this strip, the duration is 0.08 second.
T wave: indiscernible
QT interval: not measurable

Junctional rhythm

This arrhythmia occurs in the AV junctional tissue, producing retrograde depolarization of the atrial tissue and antegrade depolarization of the ventricular tissue. A junctional rhythm results from conditions that depress SA node function, such as an inferior wall MI, digitalis toxicity, and vagal stimulation. The arrhythmia may also stem from increased automaticity of the junctional tissue, which can be brought about by digitalis toxicity or ischemia associated with an inferior wall MI.

A junctional rhythm with a ventricular rate of 60 to 100 beats/minute is known as an accelerated junctional rhythm. If the ventricular rate exceeds 100 beats/minute, the arrhythmia is called junctional tachycardia. (See *Understanding types of junctional rhythm.*)

Assessment findings
The patient will have a slow pulse rate with a regular rhythm. He may be asymptomatic, or he may show signs and symptoms of decreased cardiac output, such as hypotension, syncope, and blurred vision.

Intervention
Treatment aims to identify and manage the arrhythmia's primary cause. Most patients with junctional rhythm tolerate the rhythm disturbance well and don't require direct intervention.

If the patient is symptomatic, treatment may include atropine to increase the sinus or junctional rate. Or the doctor may insert a pacemaker to maintain an effective heart rate.

Lead II

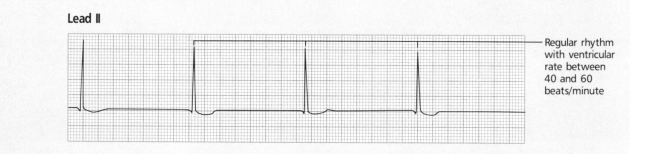

Regular rhythm with ventricular rate between 40 and 60 beats/minute

Characteristics and interpretation
Atrial rhythm: regular
Ventricular rhythm: regular
Atrial rate: if discernible, 40 to 60 beats/minute. On this strip, the rate isn't discernible.
Ventricular rate: 40 to 60 beats/minute. On this strip, the rate is 40 beats/minute.

P wave: usually inverted; may precede, follow, or fall within the QRS complex; may be absent. On this strip, the P wave is absent.
PR interval: if the P wave precedes the QRS complex, the PR interval will be less than 0.12 second and constant; otherwise it can't be measured. On this strip, it can't be measured.

QRS complex: duration within normal limits; configuration usually normal. On this strip, the duration is 0.08 second.
T wave: usually normal configuration
QT interval: usually within normal limits. On this strip, the duration is 0.32 second.

Understanding types of junctional rhythm

The ECG strips shown below pinpoint the features that characterize two types of junctional rhythm: accelerated junctional rhythm and junctional tachycardia.

Accelerated junctional rhythm
An ectopic rhythm, an accelerated junctional rhythm originates in the junctional tissue or bundle of His. The impulses control the ventricular rate at 60 to 100 beats/minute, which exceeds the rate of the junctional pacemaker.

Lead MCL₁

Absent P wave

Regular rhythm with rate between 60 and 100 beats/minute

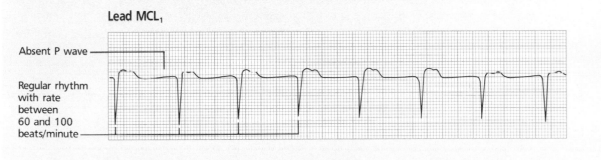

Junctional tachycardia
In junctional tachycardia, an ectopic impulse originating in the bundle of His controls ventricular contractions at a rate exceeding 100 beats/minute. Usually, the rate falls between 100 and 180 beats/minute.

Lead II

Regular rhythm with rate between 100 and 180 beats/minute

P wave follows QRS complex

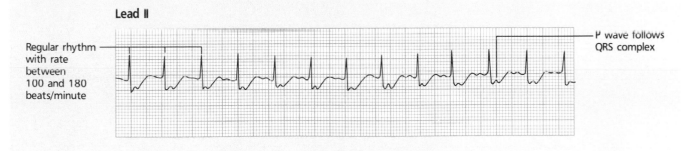

Premature junctional contractions

In premature junctional contractions (PJCs), a junctional beat occurs before the next normal sinus beat. Ectopic beats, PJCs commonly result from increased automaticity in the bundle of His or the surrounding junctional tissue, which interrupts the underlying rhythm.

PJCs most commonly result from digitalis toxicity. Their other causes include ischemia associated with an inferior wall MI, excessive caffeine ingestion, and excessive levels of amphetamines.

Assessment findings
The patient may complain of palpitations if PJCs are frequent.

Intervention
In most cases, treatment is directed at the underlying cause.

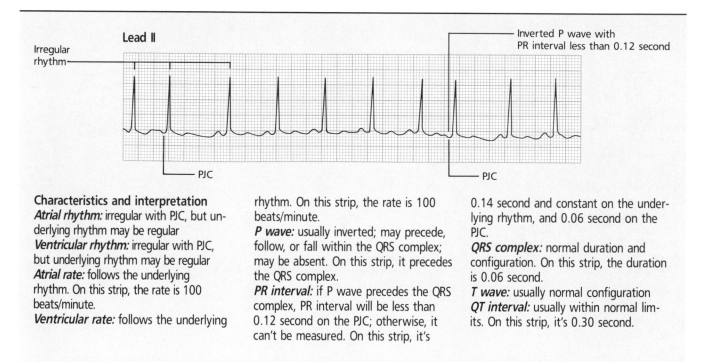

Lead II

Irregular rhythm

Inverted P wave with PR interval less than 0.12 second

PJC

PJC

Characteristics and interpretation
Atrial rhythm: irregular with PJC, but underlying rhythm may be regular
Ventricular rhythm: irregular with PJC, but underlying rhythm may be regular
Atrial rate: follows the underlying rhythm. On this strip, the rate is 100 beats/minute.
Ventricular rate: follows the underlying rhythm. On this strip, the rate is 100 beats/minute.
P wave: usually inverted; may precede, follow, or fall within the QRS complex; may be absent. On this strip, it precedes the QRS complex.
PR interval: if P wave precedes the QRS complex, PR interval will be less than 0.12 second on the PJC; otherwise, it can't be measured. On this strip, it's 0.14 second and constant on the underlying rhythm, and 0.06 second on the PJC.
QRS complex: normal duration and configuration. On this strip, the duration is 0.06 second.
T wave: usually normal configuration
QT interval: usually within normal limits. On this strip, it's 0.30 second.

Premature ventricular contractions

Among the most common arrhythmias, premature ventricular contractions (PVCs) occur in both healthy and diseased hearts. These ectopic beats may occur singly or in clusters of two or more. They also occur in bigeminy.

The many possible causes of PVCs include the use of cardiac glycosides and sympathomimetic drugs; electrolyte imbalances, such as hypokalemia and hypocalcemia; exercise; ingestion of caffeine, tobacco, or alcohol; hypoxia; MI; and myocardial irritation by pacemaker electrodes.

Complex PVCs can increase the risk of ventricular tachycardia and ventricular fibrillation.

Assessment findings
When palpating the peripheral pulse, you may feel a longer than normal pause immediately after the PVC, depending on how early in the cardiac cycle the beat occurs. The earlier the beat, the shorter the diastolic filling time, and the lower the stroke volume. Some patients complain of palpitations with frequent PVCs.

Intervention
Treatment depends on the cause of the PVCs. If the PVCs are thought to result from a cardiac problem, the doctor will order a drug, such as lidocaine, to suppress ventricular irritability. Other antiarrhythmics, such as procainamide and quinidine, may also be given.

When a patient's PVCs are thought to result from a noncardiac problem, treatment aims at correcting the underlying cause. This may mean correcting an acid-base or electrolyte disturbance, discontinuing an antiarrhythmic that's being given to treat ventricular ectopy, or treating hypothermia or correcting high catecholamine levels following open-heart surgery.

Lead MCL₁

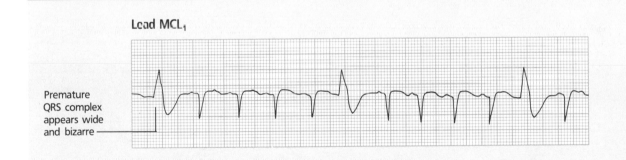

Premature QRS complex appears wide and bizarre ⎯

Characteristics and interpretation
Atrial rhythm: irregular during PVC; underlying rhythm may be regular.
Ventricular rhythm: irregular during PVC; underlying rhythm may be regular.
Atrial rate: follows underlying rhythm. On this strip, it's 120 beats/minute.
Ventricular rate: follows underlying rhythm. On this strip, it's 120 beats/minute.
P wave: atrial activity is independent of the PVC; if retrograde atrial depolarization exists, a retrograde P wave will distort the ST segment of the PVC. On this strip, no P wave appears before the PVC, but one occurs with each QRS complex.
PR interval: determined by underlying rhythm; not associated with the PVC. On this strip, the underlying PR interval is 0.12 second and constant.
QRS complex: occurs earlier than expected; duration exceeds 0.12 second with bizarre configuration. May be normal in the underlying rhythm. On this strip, it's 0.08 second in the normal beats; it's bizarre and 0.12 second in the PVC.
T wave: occurs in direction opposite QRS complex; normal in the underlying complexes
QT interval: not usually measured in the PVC, but may be within normal limits with the underlying rhythm. On this strip, it's 0.28 second in the underlying rhythm.

Ventricular tachycardia

This arrhythmia develops when three or more PVCs occur in a row and the rate exceeds 100 beats/minute. It may result from enhanced automaticity or reentry within the Purkinje system.

The rapid ventricular rate reduces ventricular filling time, and because atrial kick is lost, cardiac output drops. This puts the patient at risk for ventricular fibrillation.

Ventricular tachycardia usually results from acute MI, CAD, valvular heart disease, heart failure, or cardiomyopathy. The arrhythmia can also stem from an electrolyte imbalance, such as hypokalemia, or from toxic levels of a drug, such as digitalis, procainamide, quinidine, and disopyramide.

You may detect two variations of this arrhythmia: R-on-T phenomenon and torsades de pointes. (See *Recognizing other forms of ventricular tachycardia.*)

Assessment findings

Many patients will have signs and symptoms of decreased cardiac output, such as hypotension, an absent pulse, confusion, vertigo, and syncope. Some patients tolerate this rhythm for a short time; others become unresponsive immediately.

Intervention

This rhythm often degenerates into ventricular fibrillation and cardiovascular collapse, requiring immediate intervention with cardiopulmonary resuscitation (CPR) and defibrillation. Lidocaine is usually administered immediately. If it proves ineffective, procainamide or bretylium are used instead.

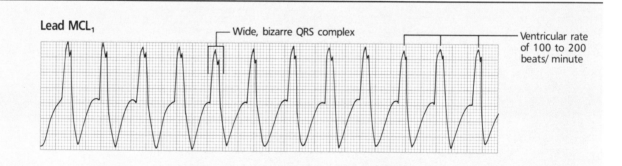

Lead MCL₁

— Wide, bizarre QRS complex

Ventricular rate of 100 to 200 beats/ minute

Characteristics and interpretation
Atrial rhythm: Independent P waves may be discernible with slower ventricular rates. On this strip, the P waves aren't visible.
Ventricular rhythm: usually regular, but may be slightly irregular. On this strip, it's regular.

Atrial rate: can't be determined
Ventricular rate: usually 100 to 200 beats/minute. On this strip, it's 120 beats/minute.
P wave: usually absent; may be obscured by the QRS complex; retrograde P waves may be present.
PR interval: not measurable

QRS complex: duration greater than 0.12 second; bizarre appearance, usually with increased amplitude. On this strip, the duration is 0.16 second.
T wave: opposite the terminal forces of the QRS complex
QT interval: not measurable

Recognizing other forms of ventricular tachycardia

Ventricular tachycardia can take two other forms—torsades de pointes and R-on-T phenomenon.

Torsades de pointes
With this arrhythmia, the ventricular rate ranges from 150 to 250 beats/minute. The rhythm is characterized by wide QRS complexes that rotate about the baseline—thus, the name, which means "twisting about the points."

Lead MCL₁

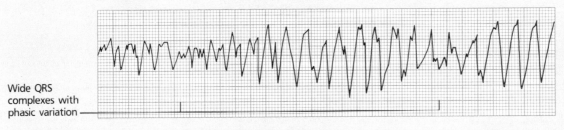

Wide QRS
complexes with
phasic variation

R-on-T phenomenon
In this arrhythmia, a PVC occurs so early in the cardiac cycle that it falls on the T wave of the previous beat. Because the cells haven't fully repolarized, ventricular tachycardia or fibrillation can occur.

Lead II

PVC on T wave
of previous beat

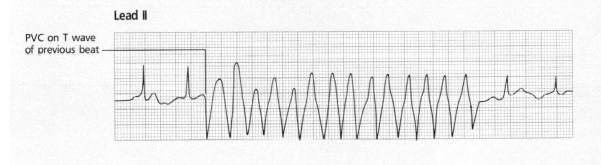

Ventricular fibrillation

Defined as chaotic asynchronous electrical activity within the ventricular tissue, ventricular fibrillation results in death if the rhythm isn't stopped immediately. Conditions leading to ventricular fibrillation include myocardial ischemia, hypokalemia, cocaine toxicity, hypoxia, hypothermia, severe acidosis, and severe alkalosis.

Patients with MIs have the greatest risk of ventricular fibrillation during the first 2 hours after the onset of chest pain. Those who experience ventricular fibrillation will have a reduced risk for recurrence as healing progresses and scar tissue forms.

Assessment findings

A lack of cardiac output results in a loss of consciousness, pulselessness, and respiratory arrest. Initially, you may see coarse fibrillatory waves on the ECG strip. As the acidosis develops, the waves become fine and progress to asystole, unless defibrillation restores cardiac rhythm.

Intervention

Perform CPR until the patient can receive defibrillation—the only effective treatment for ventricular fibrillation. Coarse fibrillation responds more quickly to defibrillation attempts. Fine fibrillation is more difficult to convert without administering epinephrine and correcting any acidosis.

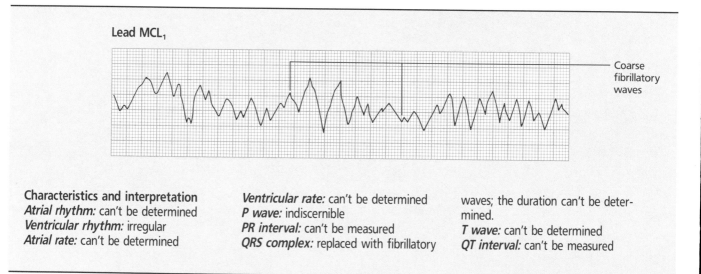

Lead MCL₁

Coarse fibrillatory waves

Characteristics and interpretation
Atrial rhythm: can't be determined
Ventricular rhythm: irregular
Atrial rate: can't be determined

Ventricular rate: can't be determined
P wave: indiscernible
PR interval: can't be measured
QRS complex: replaced with fibrillatory

waves; the duration can't be determined.
T wave: can't be determined
QT interval: can't be measured

Idioventricular rhythm

This arrhythmia acts as a safety mechanism when all potential pacemakers above the ventricles fail to discharge or when a block prevents supraventricular impulses from reaching the ventricles.

Assessment findings

The slow ventricular rate and loss of atrial kick associated with this arrhythmia will markedly reduce the patient's cardiac output. In turn, this will cause hypotension, confusion, vertigo, and syncope.

Intervention

Treatment aims to identify and manage the primary problem that triggered this safety mechanism.

Atropine may be given to increase the patient's atrial rate. A pacemaker may also be inserted to increase the heart rate and thereby improve cardiac output.

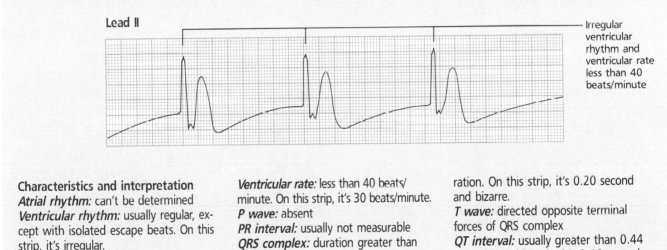

Lead II

Irregular ventricular rhythm and ventricular rate less than 40 beats/minute

Characteristics and interpretation
Atrial rhythm: can't be determined
Ventricular rhythm: usually regular, except with isolated escape beats. On this strip, it's irregular.
Atrial rate: can't be determined

Ventricular rate: less than 40 beats/minute. On this strip, it's 30 beats/minute.
P wave: absent
PR interval: usually not measurable
QRS complex: duration greater than 0.12 second; wide and bizarre configu-ration. On this strip, it's 0.20 second and bizarre.
T wave: directed opposite terminal forces of QRS complex
QT interval: usually greater than 0.44 second. On this strip, it's 0.46 second.

First-degree AV block

Defined as delayed conduction velocity through the AV node or His-Purkinje system, first-degree AV block is associated with an inferior wall MI and the effects of digitalis or amiodarone. The arrhythmia is also associated with chronic degeneration of the conduction system.

Assessment findings
Usually, patients with first-degree AV block are asymptomatic.

Intervention
Management of first-degree AV block includes identifying and treating the underlying cause, and monitoring the patient for signs of progressive AV block.

Lead II

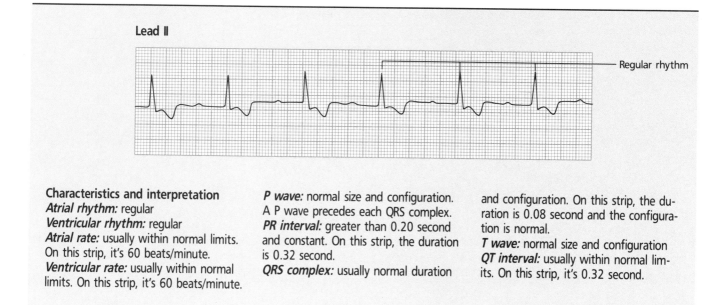

Regular rhythm

Characteristics and interpretation
Atrial rhythm: regular
Ventricular rhythm: regular
Atrial rate: usually within normal limits. On this strip, it's 60 beats/minute.
Ventricular rate: usually within normal limits. On this strip, it's 60 beats/minute.

P wave: normal size and configuration. A P wave precedes each QRS complex.
PR interval: greater than 0.20 second and constant. On this strip, the duration is 0.32 second.
QRS complex: usually normal duration

and configuration. On this strip, the duration is 0.08 second and the configuration is normal.
T wave: normal size and configuration
QT interval: usually within normal limits. On this strip, it's 0.32 second.

Type I second-degree AV block

In Type I (Wenckebach or Mobitz I) second-degree AV block, diseased AV node tissues conduct impulses to the ventricles increasingly later, until one of the atrial impulses fails to be conducted or is blocked. Type I block most commonly occurs at the level of the AV node and is caused by an inferior wall MI, vagal stimulation, or digitalis toxicity.

Assessment findings
The arrhythmia usually doesn't cause symptoms. However, a patient may have signs and symptoms of decreased cardiac output, such as hypotension, confusion, and syncope. These effects occur especially if the patient's ventricular rate is slow.

Intervention
If the patient is asymptomatic, no intervention is required, other than monitoring the ECG frequently to see if a more serious form of AV block develops.

If the patient is symptomatic, the doctor may order atropine to increase the rate and to stop the decremental conduction through the AV node. Occasionally, the doctor may insert a temporary pacemaker to maintain an effective cardiac output.

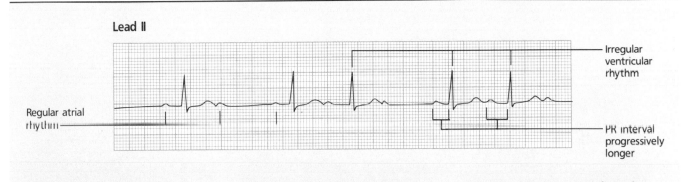

Lead II

Regular atrial rhythm

Irregular ventricular rhythm

PR interval progressively longer

Characteristics and interpretation
Atrial rhythm: regular
Ventricular rhythm: irregular
Atrial rate: determined by the underlying rhythm. On this strip, it's 80 beats/minute.
Ventricular rate: slower than the atrial rate. On this strip, it's 50 beats/minute.

P wave: normal size and configuration
PR interval: progressively prolonged with each beat until a P wave appears without a QRS complex
QRS complex: normal duration and configuration; periodically absent. On this strip, the duration is 0.08 second.

T wave: normal size and configuration
QT interval: usually within normal limits. On this strip, it's 0.46 second and constant.
Other: usually distinguished by a pattern of group beating, referred to as the footprints of Wenckebach

Type II second-degree AV block

Produced by a conduction disturbance in the His-Purkinje system, a Type II (Mobitz II) second-degree AV block causes an intermittent absence of conduction. In Type II block, two or more atrial impulses are conducted to the ventricles with constant PR intervals, when suddenly, without warning, the atrial impulse is blocked.

This type of block occurs in an anterior wall MI, severe CAD, and chronic degeneration of the conduction system.

Assessment findings

The patient's peripheral pulses may be slow and regular or irregular. If the heart rate is slow, the patient may have signs and symptoms of reduced cardiac output, including hypotension, syncope, and angina. Type II second-degree AV block frequently progresses to complete heart block with an idioventricular escape rhythm or ventricular asystole.

Intervention

If the patient is hypotensive, treatment aims at increasing his heart rate to improve cardiac output. Because the conduction block occurs in the His-Purkinje system, drugs that act directly on the myocardium usually prove more effective than those that increase the atrial rate. As a result, isoproterenol may be ordered to increase the ventricular rate instead of atropine.

If the patient has an anterior wall MI, the doctor will immediately insert a temporary pacemaker to prevent ventricular asystole. For long-term management, the patient will usually need a permanent pacemaker.

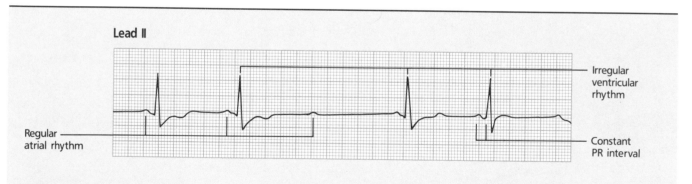

Lead II

Irregular ventricular rhythm

Regular atrial rhythm

Constant PR interval

Characteristics and interpretation
Atrial rhythm: regular
Ventricular rhythm: regular or irregular
Atrial rate: usually within normal limits. On this strip, it's 60 beats/minute.
Ventricular rate: may be within normal limits, but less than the atrial rate. On this strip, it's 40 beats/minute.

P wave: normal size and configuration. Not all P waves will be followed by a QRS complex.
PR interval: constant and frequently within normal limits for all conducted beats
QRS complex: usually greater than 0.16

second due to the presence of a preexisting bundle-branch block. On this strip, it's 0.12 second.
T wave: usually normal size and configuration
QT interval: usually within normal limits. On this strip, it's 0.44 second.

Third-degree AV block

Also called complete heart block, third-degree AV block occurs when all supraventricular impulses are prevented from reaching the ventricles. If this type of block originates at the AV node, a junctional escape rhythm occurs; if it originates below the AV node, an idioventricular escape rhythm occurs.

Third-degree AV block involving the AV node may result from an inferior wall MI or digitalis toxicity. Third-degree AV block below the AV node may result from an anterior wall MI or chronic degeneration of the conduction system.

Assessment findings
If the escape rhythm is junctional, the patient will usually maintain adequate cardiac output and thus have no signs or symptoms. Idioventricular escape rhythms, however, are slower and less stable and may produce signs and symptoms of decreased cardiac output, such as hypotension, confusion, and syncope.

Intervention
If cardiac output isn't adequate or the patient's condition seems to be deteriorating, the doctor will order therapy to improve the ventricular rhythm. Initially, atropine or isoproterenol may be ordered to increase the ventricular rate and improve cardiac output until a pacemaker can be inserted. Isoproterenol should be titrated carefully because it raises myocardial oxygen demands and places the patient at risk for developing ventricular tachycardia.

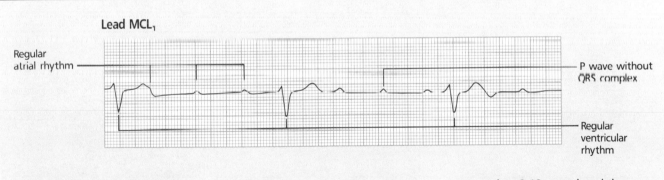

Lead MCL₁

Regular atrial rhythm

P wave without QRS complex

Regular ventricular rhythm

Characteristics and interpretation
Atrial rhythm: usually regular
Ventricular rhythm: usually regular
Atrial rate: usually within normal limits. On this strip, it's 90 beats/minute.
Ventricular rate: slow. On this strip, it's 30 beats/minute.
P wave: normal size and configuration

PR interval: can't be measured because the atria and ventricles beat independently of each other
QRS complex: determined by the site of the escape rhythm. With a junctional escape rhythm, the duration and configuration are normal; with an idioventricular escape rhythm, the duration is

greater than 0.12 second, and the complex is distorted. On this strip, the duration is 0.16 second, the configuration is abnormal, and the complex is distorted.
T wave: normal size and configuration
QT interval: may or may not be within normal limits. On this strip, it's 0.56 second.

PART 3

Interpreting
12-lead ECGs

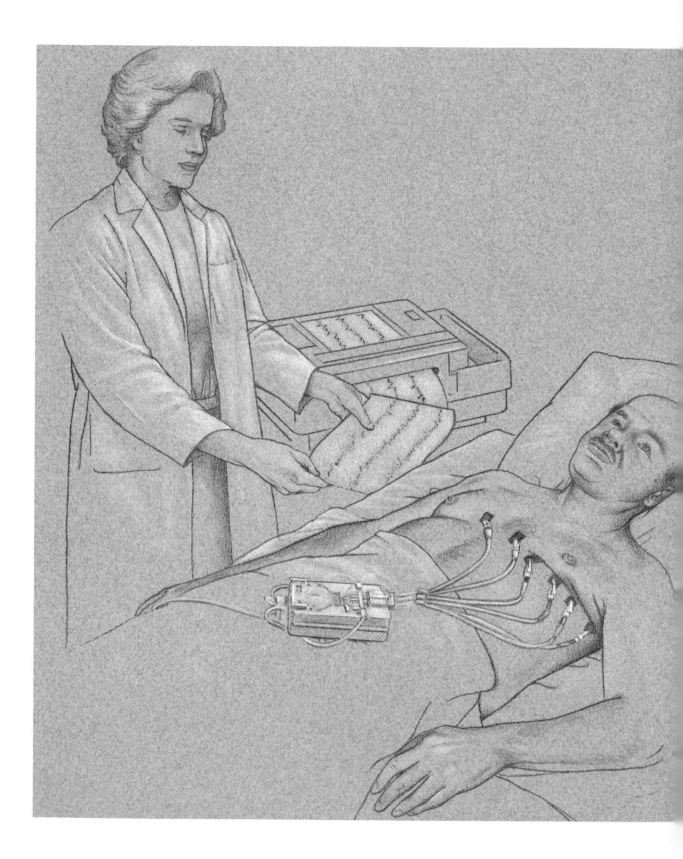

CHAPTER 5

Normal 12-lead ECG

A bedside monitor provides valuable, up-to-the-minute data about a patient's cardiac rhythm. But it can't help you identify clinical conditions, such as myocardial ischemia, myocardial injury, and heart chamber enlargement. For that, you need a 12-lead electrocardiogram (ECG), which gives you a complete picture of the heart's electrical activity.

Keep in mind, however, that a 12-lead ECG, like any diagnostic test, must be viewed in light of other clinical evidence. So always correlate your ECG findings with such information as your patient history, physical assessment findings, and the patient's medication regimen. Remember, the ECG records only the electrical events in the heart; it reveals nothing about the myocardium's ability to contract and pump blood. That's why a patient who's gravely ill with congestive heart failure may have a normal ECG, whereas a patient who's fully recovered from a myocardial infarction (MI) may have an abnormal ECG.

This chapter will help you to interpret 12-lead ECGs with confidence. The first section reviews the basic components of the 12-lead ECG, including the bipolar and unipolar limb leads, and the unipolar precordial leads. Next come thorough explanations of how to record and how to read a 12-lead ECG. The final section discusses using a signal-average ECG to avoid electrical interference.

Components of the 12-lead ECG

The 12-lead ECG provides 12 different views of the heart's electrical activity. The leads scan up, down, and across the heart, with each lead transmitting information about a particular area. That's why one lead may clearly show an abnormality that another lead omits. The 12 leads include three bipolar limb leads (I, II, and III), three unipolar augmented limb leads (aV$_R$, aV$_L$, and aV$_F$), and six unipolar precordial, or chest, leads (V$_1$, V$_2$, V$_3$, V$_4$, V$_5$, and V$_6$).

Limb leads

To record the limb leads (both bipolar and unipolar), you'll place electrodes on the patient's arms and legs. Specifically, you'll place electrodes on the right arm (RA), left arm (LA), and left leg (LL). You'll also place an electrode on the patient's right leg, but this electrode simply serves as a ground and doesn't contribute to the ECG waveform.

Bipolar limb leads

Leads I, II, and III are called bipolar because they require two electrodes—one positive and one negative. These leads record the electrical potential between the two electrodes. (See *Monitoring bipolar limb leads.*)

Usually, the QRS complex in these leads will have a positive deflection. That's because the ECG waveform always reflects the orientation of the lead to the wave of depolarization passing through the myocardium. Normally, this wave of depolarization moves through the heart from right to left and from top to bottom. Because of the positioning of the bipolar limb leads, the wave of depolarization normally moves toward the positive pole of each, creating an upright QRS complex. If, for some reason, the wave of depolarization moves toward the negative pole, the QRS complex will be deflected downward below the baseline.

Augmented limb leads

The other three limb leads have only one electrode, representing the positive pole, which makes them unipolar. The negative pole is computed by the ECG machine. Without augmentation, the tracings from these leads would be quite small. However, the ECG machine automatically enlarges (or augments) the deflections to make them more readable. This augmentation is indicated by the letter "a" on the leads aV$_R$, aV$_L$, and aV$_F$. (See *Monitoring augmented limb leads,* page 70.)

Lead aV$_R$ typically records negative QRS complex deflections because the wave of depolarization moves away from it. In lead aV$_L$, the QRS complexes are biphasic; in lead aV$_F$, they're positive.

By monitoring the heart's electrical activity from above and below, and from the right and left sides, the six limb leads give a two-dimensional view of the heart's frontal plane. Each lead scans approximately a 30-degree wedge of the heart's frontal plane. Combined, these wedges form a circle—called the hexaxial reference system—that serves as a point of reference for measuring the heart's electrical axis. (For an in-depth discussion of the hexaxial reference system and electrical axis, see Chapter 6.)

Precordial leads

To obtain a complete view of the heart's electrical activity, you'll need to examine more than the frontal plane. That's why the precordial leads prove valuable. By placing electrodes at key locations across the patient's chest, you can obtain views of the heart from different angles. The precordial leads reflect the electri-

Monitoring bipolar limb leads

For the bipolar limb leads, you'll place electrodes on the patient's wrists and ankles. To visualize the portion of the heart being viewed, think of the potential as derived from the roots of the limbs—for example, from the two shoulders and the left groin. In the illustrations below, RA indicates right arm; LA, left arm; RL, right leg; and LL, left leg. The plus sign (+) indicates the positive pole; the minus sign (−), the negative pole; and the G, the ground.

Lead I
This lead connects the right arm (negative pole) with the left arm (positive pole), reflecting electrical activity in the lateral portion of the heart.

Lead II
This lead connects the right arm (negative pole) with the left leg (positive pole), reflecting electrical activity in the inferior wall of the heart.

Lead III
This lead connects the left arm (negative pole) with the left leg (positive pole), reflecting electrical activity in the inferior wall of the heart.

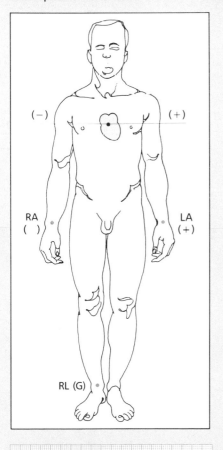

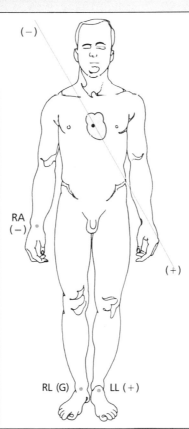

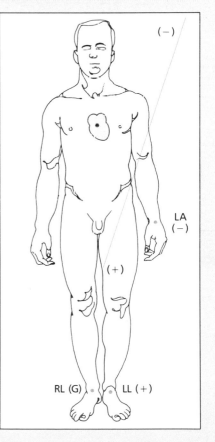

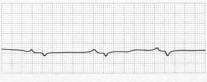

Monitoring augmented limb leads

For the augmented limb leads, you'll place electrodes as shown below. In the illustrations, RA indicates right arm; LA, left arm; and LL, left leg. The plus sign (+) indicates the positive pole; the minus sign (−), the negative pole.

Lead aV$_R$
This lead connects the right arm (positive pole) with the heart (negative pole). This lead doesn't provide a view of a specific area of the heart.

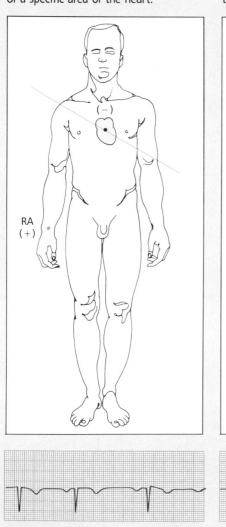

Lead aV$_L$
This lead connects the left arm (positive pole) with the heart (negative pole), providing a view of the lateral wall of the heart.

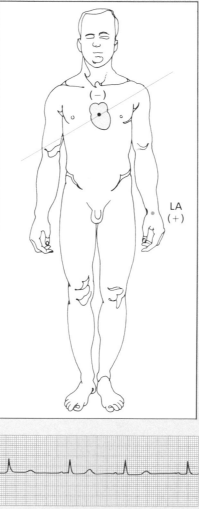

Lead aV$_F$
This lead connects the left leg (positive pole) with the heart (negative pole), providing a view of the inferior wall of the heart.

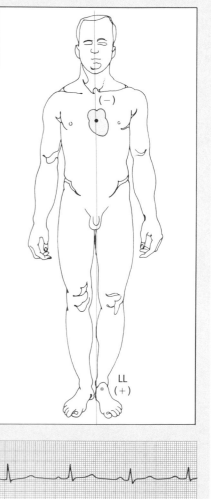

cal activity in the ventricles, on a horizontal plane.

Termed leads V_1 through V_6, these leads are unipolar, with each electrode representing the positive pole and the ECG machine computing the negative pole. To monitor these leads, you'll need to place each of the six precordial electrodes in specific locations on the patient's chest. (See *Positioning precordial electrodes*.)

Leads V_1 and V_2 typically record negative deflections of the QRS complex because the wave of depolarization moves toward the left ventricle and away from the electrodes. Because these leads monitor the right side of the heart, they're often referred to as the right precordial leads.

By contrast, leads V_3 through V_6 are called the left precordial leads. In these leads, the wave of ventricular depolarization moves toward the electrodes, creating upright, or positive, QRS complexes. In fact, the QRS complexes become progressively larger in leads V_2 through V_5 because of the positions of the corresponding electrodes. In lead V_6, the QRS complex is slightly smaller than in lead V_5.

You'll also note that the S wave is deep in leads V_1 and V_2 and that it grows progressively smaller in leads V_3 through V_6. Normally, in lead V_3, the S wave and the R wave are about the same size. This is known as the transition. When it occurs in lead V_1 or V_2, it's called an early transition; when it occurs in lead V_4, V_5, or V_6, it's called a late transition.

Complete view

By reviewing the ECG tracings from the bipolar limb leads, the augmented limb leads, and the precordial leads, you can obtain a fairly complete view of the electrical activity in the inferior, anterior, and lateral portions of the heart.

Often, the leads are grouped together and called either inferior leads, anterior leads, or lateral leads, based on the area they scan. The inferior leads are leads II, III, and aV_F; the anterior leads, leads V_1, V_2, V_3, and V_4; and the lateral leads, leads I, aV_L, V_5, and V_6. Lead aV_R doesn't provide a specific view of the heart.

Positioning precordial electrodes

The precordial leads complement the limb leads to provide a complete view of the heart. To record the precordial leads, place the electrodes as follows:
V_1 — fourth intercostal space, right sternal border
V_2 — fourth intercostal space, left sternal border
V_3 — midway between V_2 and V_4
V_4 — fifth intercostal space, left midclavicular line
V_5 — fifth intercostal space, left anterior axillary line
V_6 — fifth intercostal space, left midaxillary line

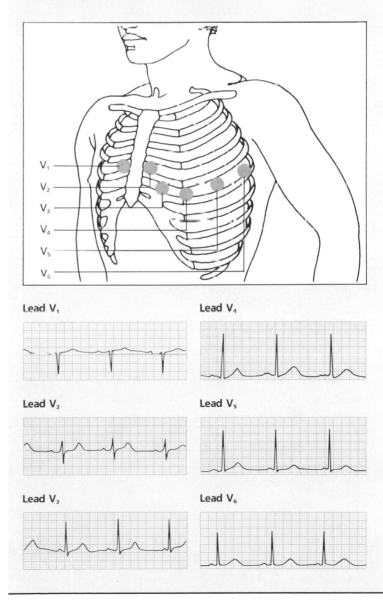

Lead V_1

Lead V_4

Lead V_2

Lead V_5

Lead V_3

Lead V_6

Recording a 12-lead ECG

You can obtain a 12-lead electrocardiogram (ECG) using either a multichannel or a single-channel ECG machine. Typically, you'll use a multichannel machine. To record your patient's 12-lead ECG using this machine, perform the procedure that follows.

Place the ECG machine close to the patient's bed, and plug the cord into the wall outlet. If the patient is already connected to a cardiac monitor, remove the electrodes to accommodate the precordial leads and minimize electrical interference on the ECG tracing. If possible, keep the patient away from electrical fixtures and power cords.

As you set up the machine, explain the procedure to the patient. Tell him that the test records the heart's electrical activity and that it may be repeated at certain intervals. Emphasize that no electrical current will enter his body. Also, tell him that the test typically takes about 5 minutes.

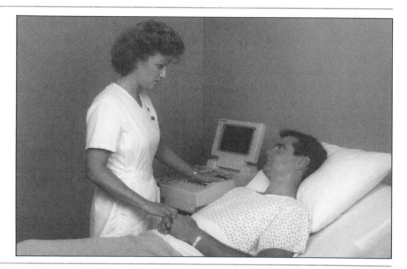

Have the patient lie supine in the center of the bed with his arms at his sides. You may raise the head of the bed to promote his comfort. Expose his arms and legs, and drape him appropriately. His arms and legs should be relaxed to minimize muscle trembling, which can cause electrical interference.

If the bed is too narrow, place the patient's hands under his buttocks to prevent muscle tension. Also use this technique if the patient is shivering or trembling. Make sure his feet aren't touching the bed board.

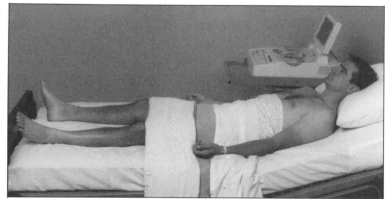

Select flat, fleshy areas to place the electrodes. Avoid muscular and bony areas. If the patient has an amputated limb, choose a site on the stump.

If an area is excessively hairy, shave it. Clean excess oil or other substances from the skin to enhance electrode contact.

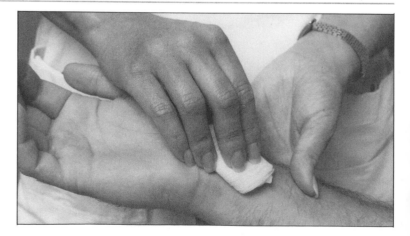

Apply the electrode paste or gel or the disposable electrodes to the patient's wrists and to the medial aspects of his ankles. If you're using paste or gel, rub it into the skin. If you're using disposable electrodes, peel off the contact paper and apply them directly to the prepared site, as recommended by the manufacturer's instructions. To guarantee the best connection to the leadwire, position disposable electrodes on the legs with the lead connection pointing superiorly.

If you're using paste or gel, secure electrodes promptly after you apply the conductive medium. This prevents drying of the medium, which could impair ECG quality.

Never use alcohol or acetone pads in place of the electrode paste or gel because they impair electrode contact with the skin and diminish the transmission quality of electrical impulses.

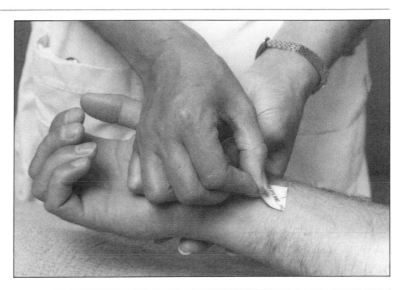

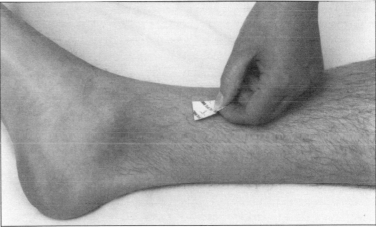

Connect the limb leadwires to the electrodes. Make sure the metal parts of the electrodes are clean and bright. Dirty or corroded electrodes prevent a good electrical connection.

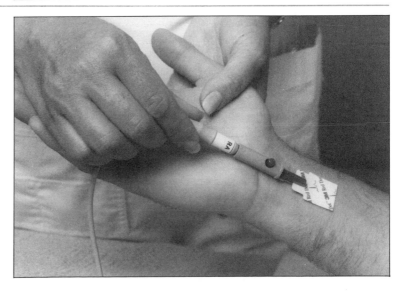

You'll see that the tip of each leadwire is lettered and color coded for easy identification. The white or RA leadwire goes to the right arm; the green or RL leadwire, to the right leg; the red or LL leadwire, to the left leg; the black or LA leadwire, to the left arm; and the brown or V_1 to V_6 leadwire, to the chest.

Now, expose the patient's chest. Put a small amount of electrode gel or paste or a disposable electrode at each electrode position. If your patient is a woman, be sure to place the chest electrodes below the breast tissue. In a large-breasted woman, you may need to displace the breast tissue laterally.

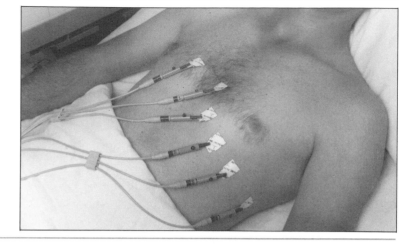

Check to see that the paper speed selector is set to the standard 25 mm/second and that the machine is set to full voltage. The machine will record a normal standardization mark—a square that's the height of two large squares or 10 small squares on the recording paper. Then, if necessary, enter the appropriate patient identification data.

If, when you record the ECG, any part of the waveform extends beyond the paper, adjust the normal standardization to half standardization. Note on the ECG that this has been done, as this will need to be considered in its interpretation.

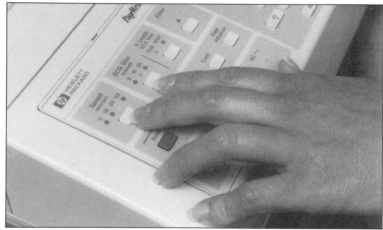

Now, you're ready to begin the recording. Ask the patient to relax and breathe normally. Tell him to lie still and not to talk when you record his ECG. Then press the "auto" button. Observe the tracing quality. The machine will record all 12 leads automatically, recording three consecutive leads simultaneously. Some machines have a display screen so you can preview waveforms before the machine records them on paper.

When the machine finishes recording the 12-lead ECG, remove the electrodes and clean the patient's skin. After disconnecting the leadwires from the electrodes, dispose of or clean the electrodes, as indicated. Record the date, time, patient's name, and room number on the ECG itself. Note any appropriate clinical information on the ECG.

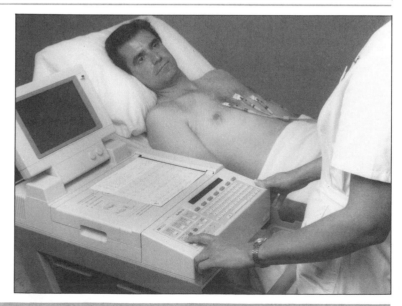

Reading a 12-lead ECG

After you've recorded a 12-lead ECG, you need to interpret your findings. To do so, follow these steps:
• First, check to make sure the ECG is technically accurate. Is the baseline free from electrical interference and drift? Does the waveform for lead aV_R deflect downward? If the answer to either of these questions is no, record another ECG.
• Next, locate the lead markers, the short vertical marks on the waveforms that indicate a change from one lead to another.
• Then, look for calibration or standardization markings to ensure that all leads were re-

Evaluating a normal 12-lead ECG

A normal 12-lead electrocardiogram (ECG), such as the one shown here, has the following characteristics:
• P waves. Deflection is usually positive but may be diphasic or inverted in leads III, aV_L, and V_1, and may be inverted in aV_R.
• PR intervals. Duration is constant in all leads.
• QRS complexes. Deflection changes with the lead, but duration remains constant.
• ST segments. Deflection is isoelectric or with minimal deviation.
• T waves. Deflection should be upright in most leads. It is inverted in lead aV_R. Occasionally, deflection is biphasic or inverted in leads III, aV_L, and V_1.

Lead I

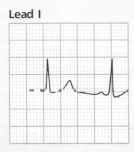

Lead aV_R

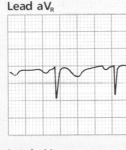

Lead V₁

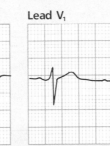

Lead V₄

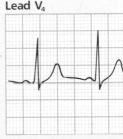

Lead II

Lead aV_L

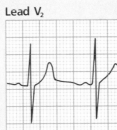

Lead V₂

Lead V₅

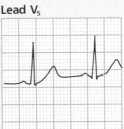

Lead III

Lead aV_F

Lead V₃

Lead V₆

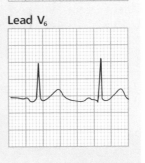

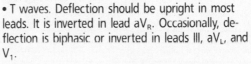

Performing a signal-average ECG

To perform a signal-average electrocardiogram (ECG), you'll need a computerized ECG machine. The unit is portable so you can run the test at the patient's bedside. Before running the test, place the patient in the supine position. Explain the importance of remaining still during the test and tell him that the test is painless and takes about 15 minutes.

Next, make sure the patient's skin in the areas of electrode placement is clean. This will help ensure good electrode contact and a minimum of interference. You'll only attach electrodes at appropriate spots on the anterior and posterior thorax. Again remind the patient to remain still. Then, begin recording. Record between 150 and 300 beats. After the test is run, feed the information into the computer.

corded using the same amplitude.

• Next, focusing on the lead II tracing, assess the heart rhythm.

• Using the quadrant method, observe the waveforms for leads I and aV$_F$. What is the heart's electrical axis? For more information about using the quadrant method or computing the electrical axis, see Chapter 6.

• Now evaluate the limb leads, looking first at leads I and II. The R wave should be taller in lead II than it is in lead I. Next, examine lead III. Typically, the tracing in this lead is similar to the tracing in lead I, but smaller. The P wave or QRS complex may be inverted. Check all of these lead tracings to make sure that the ST segments are flat, the T waves are upright, and the Q waves are absent.

• Move on to lead aV$_R$, keeping in mind that it's simply a reference lead and has no diagnostic value. Check that the P wave, the QRS complex, and the T wave are deflected downward.

• Then, examine the tracings from leads aV$_L$ and aV$_F$. These two tracings should appear similar, except that the P waves and R waves will typically appear taller in lead aV$_F$.

• Next, evaluate the precordial leads. Starting with V$_1$, note the short R wave and deep S wave. Scan the rest of the precordial tracings, moving from V$_2$ through V$_6$. You should note that the R wave increases in height until V$_5$, then gets slightly smaller in V$_6$. The deep S wave normally disappears in V$_4$ or V$_5$. To avoid confusing deep S waves with deep Q waves, carefully review all parts of the QRS complex, one part at a time. (See *Evaluating a normal 12-lead ECG*, page 75.)

Electrical interference

To understand the 12-lead ECG fully, you need to recognize its margin for error. While the machine monitors the heart's electrical activity, it may also pick up electrical activity from other sources, such as skeletal and respiratory muscles. Other sources of electrical interference include high-frequency power lines, electrodes, and amplifiers.

While modern ECG machines can override the interference from electrical equipment and power lines, they're powerless against interference from muscles. For most patients, this doesn't present a significant problem. The changes are slight and don't hinder diagnosis. Occasionally, however, the extra signals generated by the muscles may mask subtle changes in the ECG. As a result, you and the patient's doctor or nurse practitioner won't have a complete picture of the patient's cardiac status, perhaps resulting in a misdiagnosis.

For example, in patients with ischemic heart disease, the ECG may pick up muscle signals which, although barely detectable, may mask low-amplitude, high-frequency ECG waveforms that signal the patient's risk for sudden cardiac death. Known as late potentials, these waveforms occur at the end of, or immediately following, the QRS complex and last 20 to 60 milliseconds into the ST segment. Because the ST segment should remain flat, or isoelectric, any detectable activity during this time strongly suggests an electrically unstable heart, and the patient would be at significant risk for developing ventricular tachycardia.

Signal-average ECGs

By using a signal-average ECG, you can avoid such interference problems. This test involves transferring ECG impulses into a computer, which averages the waveforms into one complex. In the process, the computer amplifies the voltage of the QRS complexes as much as 1,000 times, and sometimes more. (See *Performing a signal-average ECG.*)

Once the computer has received all of the necessary impulses, it notes the number of normal QRS complexes. It then identifies a QRS complex representative of the average complex. Through this process, skeletal muscle noise becomes apparent because the timing for muscle activity is different from the timing for ventricular activity.

After the test, a cardiologist will review and interpret the final tracing. If the doctor detects low-amplitude late potentials, you'll know that the patient is at risk for sudden cardiac death.

Of course, even if the results of the test are negative, you can't completely rule out the possibility of sudden cardiac death. Other conditions that may contribute to such an occurrence include a previous MI, a history of sudden cardiac death with resuscitation, structural cardiac defects (particularly left ventricular hypertrophy), hypokalemia, and hypomagnesemia.

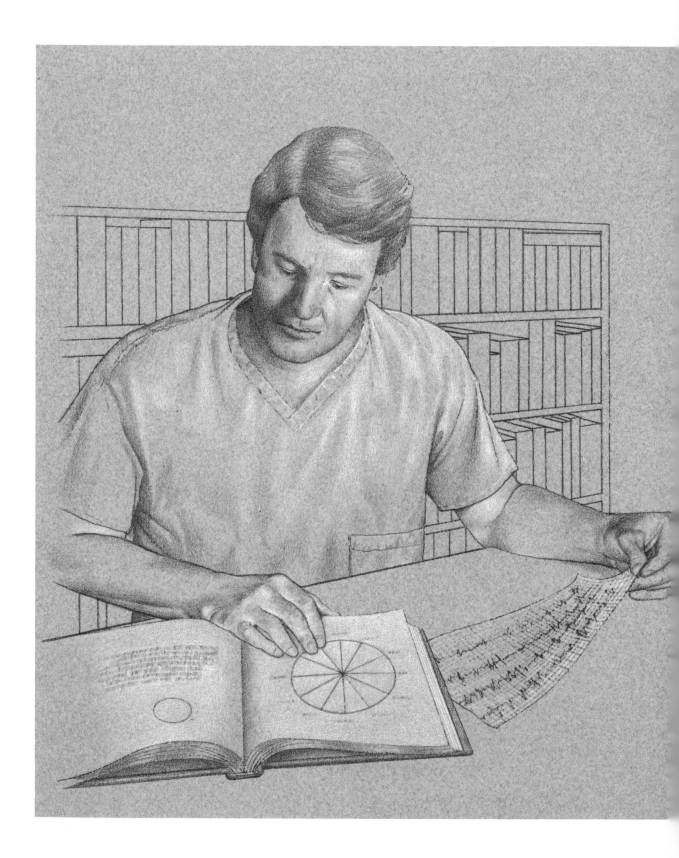

6

CHAPTER

Electrical axis determination

Why is the 12-lead electrocardiogram (ECG) such a valuable diagnostic tool?

To answer this question, first consider that a 12-lead ECG can help you identify the direction of the heart's electrical axis. And knowing the direction of this axis tells you whether or not the heart is depolarizing normally. If it isn't, electrical axis determination can also help you identify the underlying cause.

This chapter begins with an explanation of the electrical axis. Next comes information on analyzing a patient's electrical axis, including discussions of the hexaxial reference system, the quadrant method, and the degree method. The chapter concludes with a brief review of some common causes of axis deviation.

ECG limb leads: A closer look

The electrocardiogram's (ECG's) six limb leads view the heart from six different angles. This chart shows the direction of each lead relative to the wave of depolarization (shown in color) and lists the six views of the heart revealed by these leads.

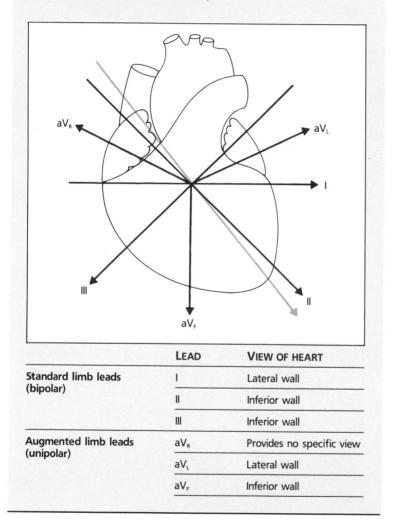

	LEAD	VIEW OF HEART
Standard limb leads (bipolar)	I	Lateral wall
	II	Inferior wall
	III	Inferior wall
Augmented limb leads (unipolar)	aV$_R$	Provides no specific view
	aV$_L$	Lateral wall
	aV$_F$	Inferior wall

Electrical axis direction

As electrical impulses travel through the heart, they generate small electrical forces called *instant-to-instant vectors*. The mean of these vectors represents the direction and force of the wave of depolarization—also known as the heart's electrical axis.

In a healthy heart, the wave of depolarization originates in the sinoatrial node, travels through the atria, the atrioventricular node, and on to the ventricles. So the normal movement is downward and to the left—the direction of a normal electrical axis.

In an unhealthy heart, the wave of depolarization (or the direction of the electrical axis) will vary. That's because the direction of electrical activity swings away from areas of damage or necrosis.

To determine the direction of your patient's electrical axis, you can use the quadrant method or the degree method. But before you use either, you need to understand the hexaxial reference system—a schematic view of the heart that uses the six limb leads.

As you know, these leads include the three standard limb leads (I, II, and III), which are bipolar, and the three augmented limb leads (aV$_R$, aV$_L$, and aV$_F$), which are unipolar. Combined, these leads give a view of the wave of depolarization in the frontal plane, including the right, left, inferior, and superior portions of the heart. (See *ECG limb leads: A closer look*.)

Hexaxial reference system

The axes of the six limb leads also make up the hexaxial reference system, which divides the heart into six equal areas. To use the hexaxial reference system, picture in your mind the position of each lead: Lead I connects the right arm (negative pole) with the left arm (positive pole); lead II connects the right arm (negative pole) with the left leg (positive pole); and lead III connects the left arm (negative pole) with the left leg (positive pole). The augmented limb leads have only one electrode, which represents the positive pole. As a result, lead aV$_R$ goes from the heart toward the right arm (positive pole); aV$_L$ goes from the heart toward the left arm (positive pole); and aV$_F$ goes from the heart to the left leg (positive pole).

Now, take this mental picture one step further and draw an imaginary line to illustrate the axis of each lead. For example, for lead I, you'd draw a horizontal line between the right and left arms; for lead II, between the right arm and left leg; and so on. All of the lines should intersect near the center, somewhere over the heart. If you draw a circle to represent the heart, you'd end up with a rough pie shape, with each wedge representing a portion of the heart monitored by each lead. (See *Understanding the hexaxial reference system.*)

This schematic representation of the heart allows you to plot your patient's electrical axis, using either the quadrant method or the degree method. If his axis falls in the right lower quadrant, between 0 degrees and +90 degrees, it's considered normal. An axis between +90 degrees and +180 degrees indicates right axis deviation; one between 0 degrees and −90 degrees, left axis deviation; and one between −180 degrees and −90 degrees, extreme axis deviation (sometimes called the northwest axis). Some experts, however, feel that the portion from 0 degrees to −30 degrees has no clinical significance.

Quadrant method
A simple, rapid method for determining the heart's axis is the quadrant method, in which you observe the main deflection of the QRS complex in leads I and aV_F. The QRS complex serves as the traditional marker for determining the electrical axis because the ventricles produce the greatest amount of electrical force when they contract. Lead I will indicate whether impulses are moving to the right or left; lead aV_F, whether they're moving up or down. (See *Using the quadrant method*, page 82.)

On the waveform for lead I, a positive main deflection of the QRS complex indicates that the electrical impulses are moving to the right, toward the positive pole of the lead, which is at the 0-degree position on the hexaxial reference system. Conversely, a negative deflection indicates that the impulses are moving to the left, toward the negative pole of the lead,

Understanding the hexaxial reference system

The hexaxial reference system consists of six bisecting lines, each representing one of the six limb leads, and a circle, representing the heart. The intersection of all of these lines divides the circle into equal, 30-degree segments.

Note that 0 degrees appears at the 3 o'clock position. Moving counterclockwise, the degrees become increasingly negative, until reaching ∓180 degrees at the 9 o'clock position. The bottom half of the circle contains the corresponding positive degrees. A positive-degree designation doesn't necessarily mean that the pole is positive.

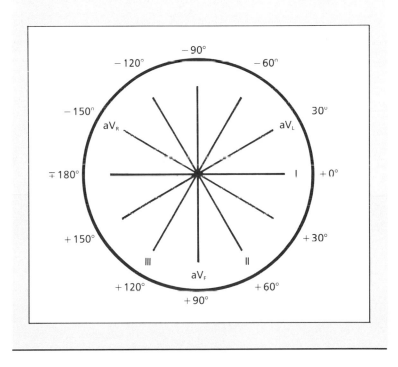

which is at the ∓180-degree position on the hexaxial reference system.

On the waveform for lead aV_F, a positive deflection of the QRS complex indicates that the electrical impulses are traveling downward,

Using the quadrant method

This chart can help you quickly determine the direction of a patient's electrical axis, which is indicated by the colored arrow. Just observe the deflections of the QRS complexes in leads I and aV$_F$. Then check the chart to determine if the patient's axis is normal or if it has a left, right, or extreme deviation.

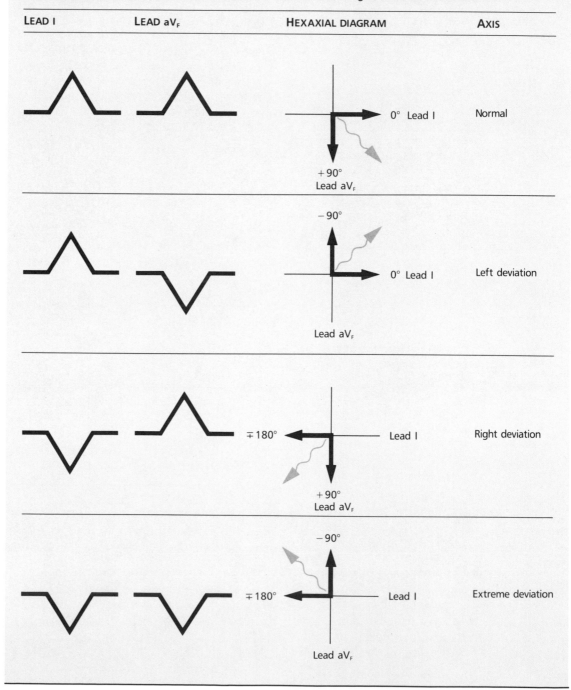

toward the positive pole of the lead, which is at the +90-degree position of the hexaxial reference system. A negative deflection indicates that impulses are traveling upward, toward the negative pole of the lead, which is at the −90-degree position of the hexaxial reference system.

Plotting this information on the hexaxial reference system (with the horizontal axis representing lead I and the vertical axis representing lead aV_F) will reveal the patient's electrical axis. For example, if lead I shows a positive deflection of the QRS complex, darken the horizontal axis between the center of reference system and the 0-degree position. If lead aV_F also shows a positive deflection of the QRS complex, darken the vertical axis between the center of reference system and the +90-degree position. The quadrant between the two axes you've darkened indicates the patient's electrical axis. In this case, it's the left lower quadrant, which indicates a normal electrical axis.

Degree method

A more precise axis calculation technique is the degree method. This method not only gives an exact degree measurement of the electrical axis — instead of simply isolating the axis between, say, 0 degrees and −90 degrees — but it also allows you to determine a patient's electrical axis even if the QRS complex is neither clearly positive nor clearly negative in leads I and aV_F.

The first step in using the degree method is to review all six leads and identify the one that contains either the smallest QRS complex, or the QRS complex that has an equal deflection above and below the baseline (equiphasic). The next step is to use the hexaxial diagram to identify the lead perpendicular to this lead. For example, if the lead with the smallest QRS complex is lead I, the lead perpendicular to the line representing lead I would be aV_F.

After you've identified the perpendicular lead, examine its QRS complex. If it's above the baseline, you know that the current is moving toward the positive pole; if the QRS complex is below the baseline, the current is moving toward the negative pole. By plotting this information on the hexaxial diagram, you can determine the direction of the electrical axis. (See *Using the degree method*, page 84, and *Finding the degree: A quick way*, page 85.)

Causes of axis deviation

Determining a patient's electrical axis can help confirm a diagnosis or narrow the range of clinical possibilities. Many factors influence the electrical axis, including the position of the heart within the chest, the size of the heart, the conduction pathways, and the force of electrical generation.

As you know, cardiac electrical activity swings away from areas of damage or necrosis. More specifically, electrical forces in the healthy portion of the heart take over for weak, or even absent, electrical forces in the damaged portion. For instance, after an inferior wall myocardial infarction, portions of the inferior wall can no longer conduct electricity. As a result, the major electrical vectors shift to the left, resulting in a left axis deviation.

Typically, the damaged portion of the heart is the last area to be depolarized. For example, in a left anterior hemiblock, the left anterior fascicle of the left bundle branch can no longer conduct electricity. Therefore, the portion normally served by the left bundle branch is the last portion of the heart to be depolarized. This shifts electrical forces to the left; consequently, the ECG will show left axis deviation.

An opposite shift occurs with right bundle-branch block. In this condition, the wave of impulse travels quickly down the normal left side, but much more slowly down the damaged right side. This shifts the electrical forces to the right, causing a right axis deviation.

An axis shift also takes place when the right or left ventricle is being paced artificially. It likewise takes place when the ventricles are

Using the degree method

The degree method, which consists of three steps, allows you to identify a patient's electrical axis by degrees on the hexaxial system, not just by the quadrant.

Step 1
Identify the lead with the smallest QRS complex or the equiphasic QRS complex. In this example, it's lead III.

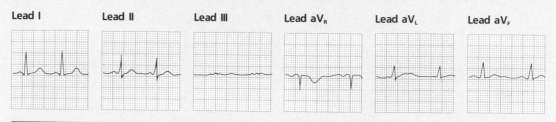

| Lead I | Lead II | Lead III | Lead aV$_R$ | Lead aV$_L$ | Lead aV$_F$ |

Step 2
Locate the axis for lead III on the hexaxial diagram. Then find the axis perpendicular to it, which is the axis for lead aV$_R$.

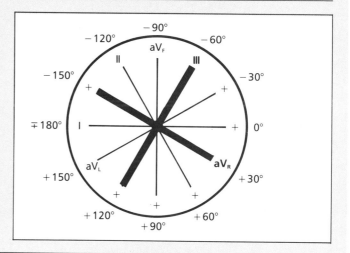

Step 3
Now, examine the QRS complex in lead aV$_R$, noting whether the deflection is positive or negative. As you can see, the QRS complex for this lead is negative. Thus, you know that the electric current is moving toward the negative pole of aV$_R$, which, on the hexaxial diagram, is in the right lower quadrant at +30 degrees. So the electrical axis in this example is normal at +30 degrees.

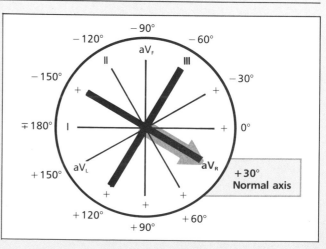

+30°
Normal axis

depolarizing abnormally, such as occurs in ventricular tachycardia. Both of these conditions can cause a left axis deviation or, occasionally, an extreme axis deviation.

Axis deviation may also result from ventricular hypertrophy. For example, an enlarged right ventricle generates greater electrical forces than normal and would consequently shift the electrical axis to the right. Wolff-Parkinson-White syndrome may produce a right, left, or extreme axis deviation, depending on which part of the ventricle is activated early.

Sometimes, axis deviation may be a normal variation, as in infants and children who normally experience right axis deviation. It may also stem from noncardiac causes. For example, if the heart is shifted in the chest cavity because of a high diaphragm from pregnancy, expect to find a left axis deviation. Also, if a patient's heart is situated on the right side of his chest instead of the left (a condition called dextrocardia), expect to find a right axis deviation.

Finding the degree: A quick way

The following chart will help you quickly identify the degree of axis deviation. After identifying the lead that contains the smallest QRS complex, consult the chart to learn which lead is perpendicular to that lead. Then check the electrocardiogram tracing for the perpendicular lead. Is the QRS complex deflected positively or negatively? If it's positive, check the column labeled "positive" to learn the electrical axis position. If it's deflected negatively, you'll find the correct axis position under the column labeled "negative."

SMALLEST QRS COMPLEX	PERPENDICULAR LEAD	POSITIVE	NEGATIVE
I	aV$_F$	+90°	−90°
II	aV$_L$	−30°	+150°
III	aV$_R$	−150°	+30°
aV$_R$	III	+120°	−60°
aV$_L$	II	+60°	−120°
aV$_F$	I	0°	∓180°

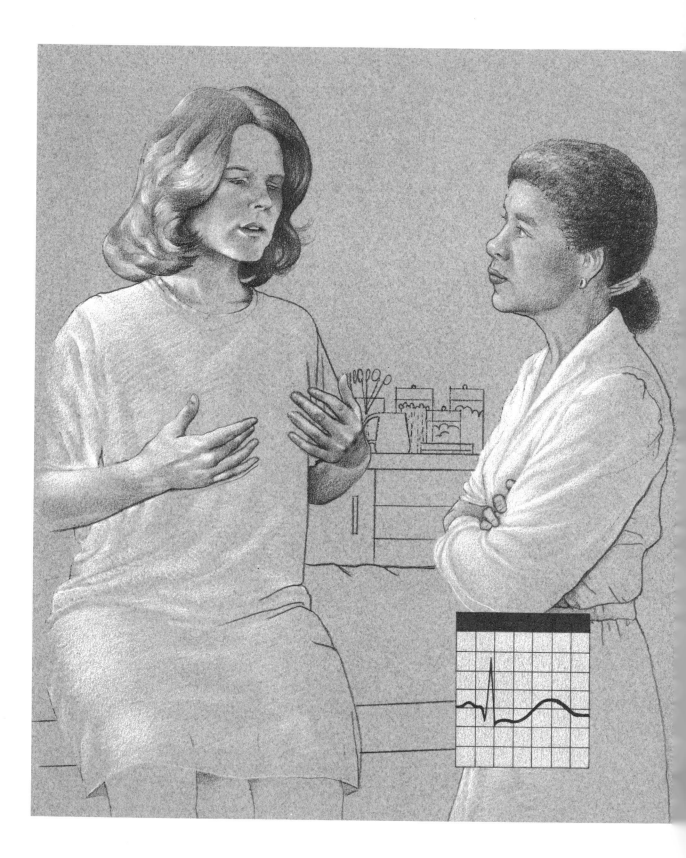

CHAPTER

Unstable angina

Caring for a patient with unstable angina requires expert electrocardiogram (ECG) interpretation skills. You must be able, for instance, to recognize the ECG changes that signal an anginal attack and to identify the changes that indicate the affected coronary artery. Identifying these ECG changes as they occur allows you to take the steps necessary to prevent a myocardial infarction (MI).

And as the bedside nurse, you're likely to be the first person to recognize and report such ECG changes. That's because they're frequently transient and can occur at any time.

Designed to help you identify characteristic ECG changes, this chapter begins by reviewing the causes of unstable angina. Then comes a section on the assessment findings you can expect when a patient experiences unstable angina. Next, the chapter covers the ECG changes most commonly seen with unstable angina, as well as the changes that help you identify which coronary artery has been oc-

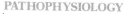

What triggers platelet aggregation

Platelets normally produce a substance called thromboxane A_2, which makes them stick together. At the same time, the endothelium of coronary vessels produces chemicals that work to prevent platelet aggregation. These include prostacyclin (PGI-2), tissue plasminogen activator (t-PA), and endothelial-derived relaxing factor (EDRF).

In patients with unstable angina, thromboxane A_2 and serotonin appear to accumulate in certain vessels, whereas the supply of PGI-2, t-PA, and EDRF declines. As a result, platelets aggregate in the coronary arteries. This temporarily cuts off blood flow, causing myocardial ischemia and the pain of an angina attack.

cluded. The last section of the chapter reviews treatments for unstable angina.

Causes

As with stable angina, unstable angina causes episodic chest pain whenever the myocardium demands more oxygen than the coronary arteries can deliver. The condition evolves primarily because the coronary arteries have become narrowed from coronary artery disease (CAD). For example, when the heart's work load increases, as during physical activity, the myocardium may demand more oxygen-rich blood than the stenotic vessels can deliver. When this occurs, the portion of the myocardium fed by a particular stenotic vessel becomes ischemic and pain results. Unlike with an MI, however, the involved tissue in unstable angina doesn't become necrotic.

Influencing factors

Several factors influence the development of unstable angina and can trigger an ischemic attack. These include the progression of ath-

erosclerosis, platelet aggregation, thrombosis, and coronary vasospasm. Although these factors often occur in combination with each other, any one may contribute to the development of unstable angina.

Progression of atherosclerosis

Many patients develop unstable angina when their CAD worsens significantly. This progression of atherosclerosis appears to affect severely stenotic vessels as well as those with minimal plaque.

Platelet aggregation

Many experts feel that patients with unstable angina experience ischemic attacks because platelets spontaneously clump together and temporarily occlude a coronary vessel — typically a vessel that's stenotic. This cuts off blood flow to an area of the myocardium, causing pain. Such episodic platelet aggregation explains why a patient with unstable angina can develop chest pain while at rest. (See *What triggers platelet aggregation.*)

Thrombosis

As with platelet aggregation, thrombosis appears to have a role in triggering unstable angina attacks. This theory evolved when doctors — performing coronary angiography and angioscopy on patients with unstable angina who were in the midst of an ischemic attack — discovered intracoronary filling defects that appeared to be caused by thrombi. After thrombolytic therapy, the patients' filling defects disappeared, the degree of coronary stenosis lessened, and the occluded arteries opened. Plus, when doctors performed autopsies on patients who'd had unstable angina, they found that the patients had been suffering from ongoing thrombosis. With this in mind, you can see why unstable angina may be prodromal to a major coronary occlusion or an acute MI.

Coronary vasospasm

Studies show that in patients with unstable angina, coronary vessels tend to experience spasm at previously injured areas. Such a spasm would, of course, cut off blood flow to the myocardium, resulting in ischemia and pain. To complicate matters, this state of hyperreactivity in the vessel seems to result in thrombi formation.

Assessment findings

Symptoms of chronic angina usually remain constant. So if a patient with chronic angina complains that his symptoms have changed or worsened, suspect unstable angina. Remember, though, that unstable angina may also develop spontaneously.

A patient with unstable angina usually reports intense chest pain, which may radiate to the left shoulder and down the inside of the left arm, or straight through to the back and into the throat, jaw, teeth, or down the right arm. The pain may occur with little or no exertion and may even awaken the patient from sleep. Attacks may last as long as 30 minutes. (Pain that lasts longer generally indicates an MI.) The patient may also complain of associated symptoms, such as nausea and diaphoresis.

During an attack, you may hear a transient systolic murmur upon auscultation. This is caused by mitral regurgitation from papillary muscle dysfunction. If the patient has left ventricular dysfunction, you may auscultate an S_3 or S_4 gallop and note a dyskinetic apical pulse. None of these heart sounds, however, are specific to angina; an MI will cause the same sounds.

An angina attack won't raise cardiac enzyme levels; that only happens if the myocardium has been damaged from an MI. Sometimes, however, severe unstable angina may resemble a small MI in both pathophysiology and prognosis.

Characteristic ECG changes

Most patients with unstable angina exhibit specific ECG changes related to ischemia only during an anginal attack. Some patients may show these changes at any time, although this usually means that another process is involved,

Monitoring the patient with unstable angina

When monitoring a patient with unstable angina, use lead V_2 or V_3. Patients with unstable angina are at risk for critical left anterior descending (LAD) stenosis (Wellens syndrome), which can affect a large area of the anterior left ventricle, possibly leading to a large anterior wall myocardial infarction. Key features of Wellens syndrome include deep, symmetrical T-wave inversion in leads V_2 and V_3 with no loss of precordial R wave. These leads show activity in the anterior wall of the left ventricle and will reflect the electrocardiogram changes that indicate stenosis of the LAD coronary artery.

Lead V_2

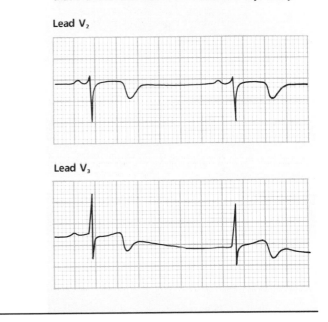

Lead V_3

such as a non–Q-wave MI. (See *Monitoring the patient with unstable angina.*)

Because characteristic ECG changes may be fleeting, you should always run a 12-lead ECG when a patient reports chest pain. All patients hospitalized with unstable angina require continuous monitoring for ECG changes, some of which require immediate intervention.

Myocardial ischemia produces two key ECG changes—ST-segment depression and an al-

Recognizing ST-segment depression

An ST segment depressed below the baseline of the electrocardiogram is a hallmark of myocardial ischemia. Be careful, though, not to confuse ST-segment depression with J-point depression, which may occur normally after exercise.

The J point is simply the junction between the QRS complex and the ST segment. When only the J point is depressed, you'll note that the ST segment starts below the baseline, but then slopes upward, as shown on the left. However, when the ST segment is truly depressed, it remains level a certain distance below the baseline, as shown on the right. With angina, the ST segment commonly remains 1 mm or more below the baseline for at least 0.08 second past the J point.

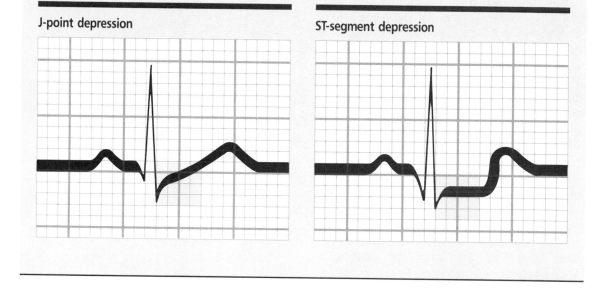

J-point depression

ST-segment depression

tered T wave—which typically occur during anginal attacks. Occasionally, you may see an elevated ST segment; this finding suggests coronary vasospasm. (See *Recognizing ST-segment depression.*)

Normally, the T wave appears slightly asymmetrical with a slow upward slope, a blunt apex, and a rapid descent. When a patient with unstable angina has an attack of chest pain, the T wave may assume a symmetrical shape, and its apex may become either peaked or flattened. The T wave will also typically invert.

Keep in mind, though, that ischemia isn't the only cause of inverted T waves. Other causes include a non-Q-wave MI, pericarditis, and left ventricular hypertrophy. Plus, patients with CAD who have a premature ventricular contraction may have an inverted T wave with the next normal complex. (See *ECG changes associated with angina.*)

Occasionally, the ECG may reveal changes associated with myocardial ischemia before the patient experiences chest pain. (This condition is known as silent ischemia.) As well, ECG findings help predict the patient's prognosis. For example, patients who show ST-segment depression or elevation are more likely to require coronary artery bypass graft (CABG) surgery, to suffer an MI, or to die, than are patients who don't show such changes.

Identifying the affected vessel

The ECG of a patient with unstable angina also helps pinpoint which coronary vessel is causing myocardial ischemia. This crucial information al-

ECG changes associated with angina

Here are some of the classic electrocardiogram (ECG) changes you may see when monitoring a patient with angina.

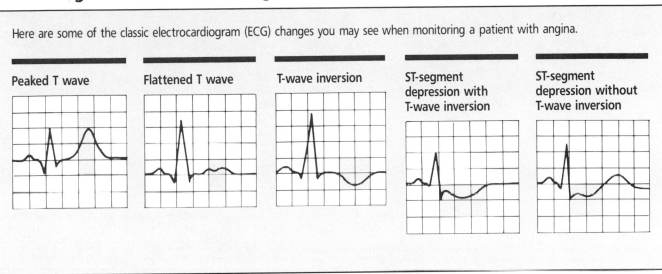

Peaked T wave   **Flattened T wave**   **T-wave inversion**   **ST-segment depression with T-wave inversion**   **ST-segment depression without T-wave inversion**

lows early detection of potentially serious conditions. For example, an occlusion of a major coronary vessel — such as the left anterior descending (LAD) or left main coronary artery — can lead to an extensive MI, profound myocardial damage, and even death. By recognizing such conditions early, you can intervene appropriately and possibly prevent the MI from occurring.

Stenosis of the LAD coronary artery
Also known as Wellens syndrome, critical stenosis high in the LAD artery impedes oxygen delivery to a large portion of the anterior left ventricle. Early recognition of characteristic ECG changes helps prevent this condition from resulting in a large anterior wall MI.

When a patient with Wellens syndrome is free from pain, you'll see deeply inverted, symmetrical T waves, which become even more deeply inverted in the precordial leads. When monitoring the patient using lead V_2 or V_3, you may notice a depressed baseline after a flattened T wave. Expect to see little or no ST-segment depression and no Q waves. When the patient is having pain, the ECG should show positive T waves with either ST-segment depression or elevation.

Usually, these ECG changes occur when the patient starts having pain and is admitted to the hospital. Sometimes, however, they don't develop until 3 to 5 days after the pain has abated. (See *Recognizing ECG changes in Wellens syndrome*, pages 92 and 93.)

Left main and triple vessel disease
Other ECG changes, particularly in the ST segment, may indicate stenosis in the left main coronary artery or triple vessel CAD. With these conditions, key ECG characteristics include ST-segment elevation in leads aV_R and V_1, and ST-segment depression in eight or more leads (with the depression most prominent in leads V_3 through V_5). Again, early detection of these ECG changes allows for timely intervention, which can prevent an MI.

The ECG changes are most apparent during episodes of chest pain. Among patients with unstable angina who have a normal ECG when asymptomatic, as many as 25% exhibit as much as a 99% stenosis of the left main coronary artery during attacks. (See *Recognizing left main coronary artery disease*, page 94.)

Recognizing ECG changes in Wellens syndrome

Some patients with Wellens syndrome experience a delay between the onset of pain and the appearance of certain electrocardiogram (ECG) changes. On this page and the next, you'll see 12-lead ECGs for a patient with Wellens syndrome. The first one was recorded while the patient was experiencing pain. Yet leads V_1, V_2, and V_3 show only slightly

negative ends on the T waves. However, in the second tracing, which was taken 12 hours later when the patient was no longer experiencing pain, leads V_2 through V_6 show deeply inverted, symmetrical T waves and ST-segment abnormalities typical of Wellens syndrome.

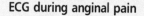

ECG during anginal pain

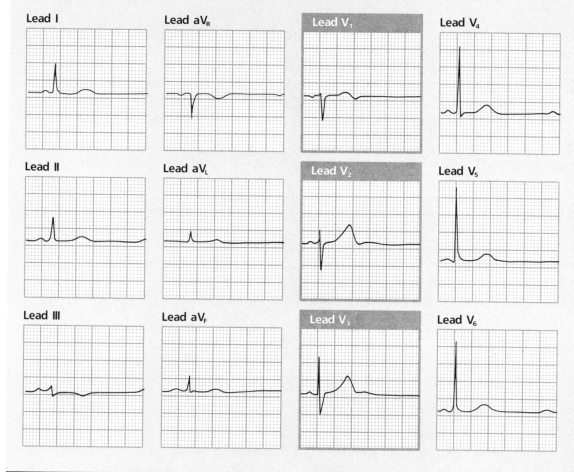

Treatment

Unstable angina is more unpredictable than chronic angina and must be treated as a medical emergency. In fact, the onset of unstable angina often portends an acute MI. Thus, be-

sides attempting to relieve the patient's pain, the main goal of treatment is to prevent sudden death. Typically, a patient suspected of having unstable angina will be hospitalized, placed on bed rest, and monitored continuously. You should ensure a calm, quiet environ-

ECG after cessation of anginal pain

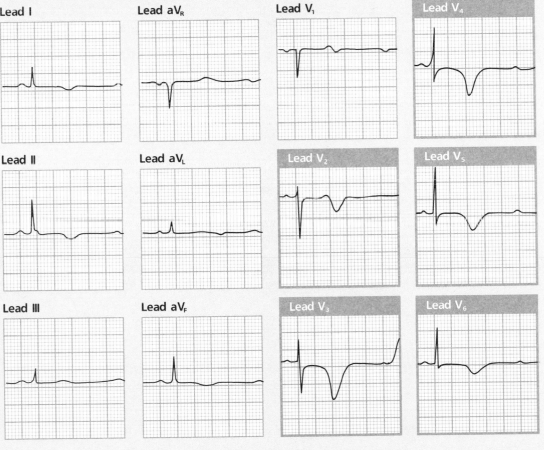

ment so the patient can receive the physical and emotional rest he needs.

The doctor will attempt to rule out an MI and other illnesses, such as pneumonia and acute GI disturbances, whose symptoms may mimic angina. As well, the diagnostic workup

will try to identify any condition that could heighten myocardial oxygen demand, such as infection, fever, thyrotoxicosis, anemia, an arrhythmia, or an exacerbation of pre-existing heart failure. Other aspects of the patient's

Recognizing left main coronary artery disease

This 12-lead electrocardiogram tracing indicates left main coronary artery disease. Note the elevation of the ST segment in leads V_1 and aV_R and the depression of the ST segment in leads V_2 through V_6 and in leads I, II, and aV_L. If you examine leads II, III, and aV_F, you'll see Q waves, indicating a previous inferior wall myocardial infarction.

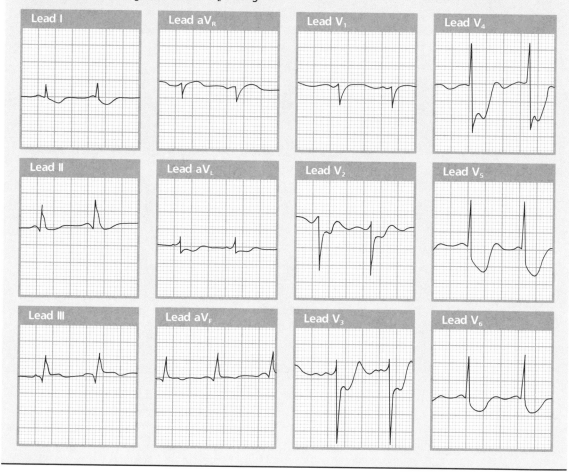

care may include medication and surgical procedures.

Drug therapy
Drugs represent a key component of the treatment for unstable angina. The most commonly prescribed drugs include nitrates, beta blockers, calcium channel blockers, and aspirin.

Nitrates
Used for more than 100 years to treat angina, nitrates work primarily by dilating veins throughout the body. In larger doses, the drug also dilates arterioles. This vasodilating effect lowers systemic vascular resistance, which helps reduce afterload and eases the heart's work load. In turn, myocardial oxygen consumption (known as MVO_2) declines and the symptoms of angina are relieved. Nitrates also dilate the coronary arteries, improving the delivery of oxygen-rich blood to the myocardium. During acute ischemic episodes, a patient may

receive nitroglycerin I.V. to maintain a constant level of the drug.

Beta blockers
Part of the sympathetic nervous system, beta receptors are scattered throughout the body. When stimulated by the release of catecholamines, beta$_1$ receptors — found primarily in the myocardium — increase the heart rate and the strength of contractions. These effects directly increase MVO$_2$. Additional beta$_1$ receptors in the kidneys trigger the release of renin, resulting in sodium and fluid retention. This retained fluid increases preload, adding to the heart's work load and further elevating MVO$_2$.

Beta blockers inhibit the effect of catecholamines on beta receptors. Therefore, the work load of the heart decreases, and MVO$_2$ declines.

Taking beta blockers alone or with nitrates may help decrease the number of ischemic episodes suffered by a patient with unstable angina and may also reduce the risk of an MI. Adding beta blockers to a regimen of nitrates and calcium channel blockers can decrease the number and duration of anginal episodes and may also help relieve silent ischemia. Even if a patient doesn't regularly take any medication for his angina, taking a beta blocker alone or in combination with nitrates or calcium channel blockers can help relieve an anginal attack.

Calcium channel blockers
These drugs stop the flow of calcium ions into cells, thereby relaxing vascular smooth muscle and preventing coronary artery vasospasm. Calcium channel blockers also dilate peripheral vessels, decreasing afterload and MVO$_2$.

Besides these actions, calcium channel blockers also reduce myocardial contractility, decreasing MVO$_2$. Because of this effect on myocardial contractility, you should give these drugs cautiously to patients with impaired left ventricular function.

Administering a calcium channel blocker along with a beta blocker can help relieve angina, delay the need for CABG surgery, reduce the risk of an MI, and even reduce the risk of death — at least on a short-term basis. A calcium channel blocker may also help prevent

anginal attacks when beta blockers and nitrates prove ineffective.

Aspirin
Aspirin prevents platelet aggregation, thus helping to ensure the patency of coronary vessels. This not only helps prevent ischemic attacks but also may reduce the patient's risk of an MI.

Procedures
The patient's doctor will consider surgery and other procedures when drug therapy fails to relieve the symptoms, or when the affected vessel requires immediate treatment. For example, a patient with Wellens syndrome who hasn't yet had an MI requires emergency cardiac catheterization and then, possibly, immediate CABG surgery.

Besides CABG, other interventions for unstable angina include angioplasty and intra-aortic balloon counterpulsation.

CABG surgery
The treatment of choice for patients with unstable angina who have multiple vessel disease and a low ejection fraction, CABG surgery can successfully reduce anginal attacks. This, in turn, can enhance the patient's quality of life.

Angioplasty
This procedure involves inserting a balloon-tipped catheter into a partially obstructed vessel and then inflating the balloon. In 90% of patients, the procedure successfully dilates the vessel. However, vessels opened through angioplasty tend to reocclude. Angioplasty also carries a greater risk for complications than does CABG surgery.

Intra-aortic balloon counterpulsation
If the patient responds poorly to medical therapy, the doctor may consider inserting an intra-aortic counterpulsating balloon. This device works to reduce systolic afterload — which decreases the work load of the heart — while increasing diastolic pressure — which enhances coronary arterial flow. This temporary measure can help relieve pain until the patient can undergo angioplasty or CABG surgery.

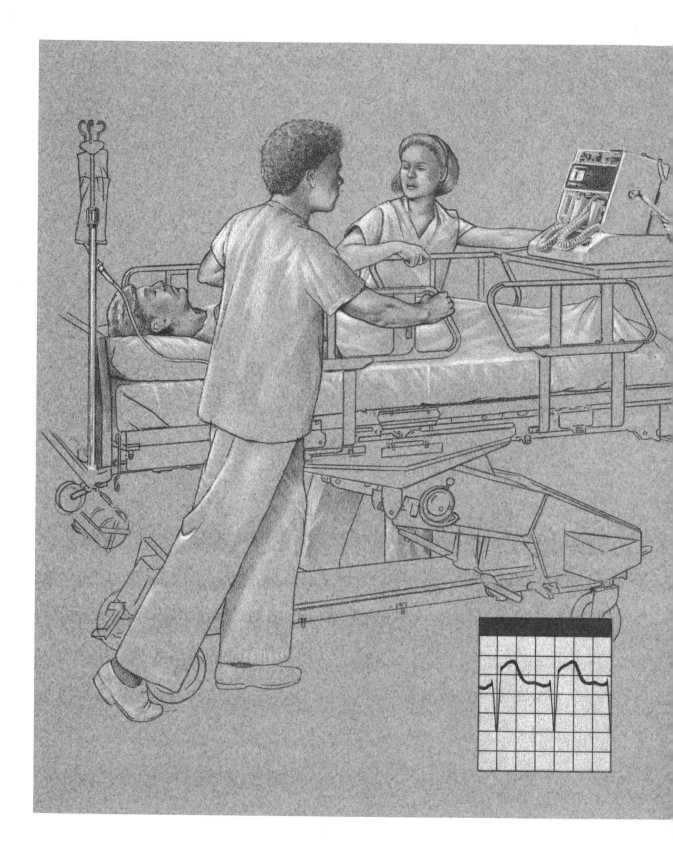

8 CHAPTER

Acute myocardial infarction

Traditionally, ischemic heart disease has been considered a male disease. But that's no longer true. Of the more than 5 million people in North America afflicted with ischemic heart disease, many now are women. In fact, the number of women with ischemic heart disease is rapidly approaching the number of men.

Whether your patient is a man or woman, detecting ischemic heart disease early can mean the difference between life and death. By recognizing characteristic electrocardiogram (ECG) changes, you may detect early ischemia, thereby allowing appropriate interventions to prevent a potentially deadly myocardial infarction (MI). And by identifying the leads in which the ECG changes occur, you can pinpoint the location of the myocardial damage.

In this chapter, you'll first review the causes of MIs. After an explanation of the typical assessment findings for an MI, the chapter focuses on the characteristic ECG changes for the three phases of an MI. Next comes a section explaining the various types of MIs and telling you how to identify them. The last two sections of the chapter cover additional diagnostic tests and treatments for MIs.

Causes

When coronary blood flow to a portion of the myocardium is reduced, ischemia develops. If the ischemia isn't relieved within 15 minutes—either by decreasing the heart's work load or by increasing the blood flow—an infarction occurs. The affected tissue becomes necrotic and eventually scars. This area of dead tissue distinguishes an MI from transient ischemia.

Clearly, any condition that causes myocardial ischemia may cause an MI. The most common cause is severe coronary artery disease (CAD), which results from progressive atherosclerosis. Other causes include platelet aggregation, thrombosis, cocaine abuse, and coronary vasospasms.

Risk factors for CAD
Many people don't know they have CAD until they experience an MI. But various risk factors can help them recognize their potential for developing CAD—and an MI. These factors include hyperlipidemia, diabetes mellitus, hypertension, stress, certain genetic factors, smoking, a sedentary life-style, and obesity.

Hyperlipidemia
High levels of cholesterol and other lipids in the bloodstream clearly contribute to atherosclerosis. Although the relationship between diet and hyperlipidemia is controversial, most studies suggest that a diet high in cholesterol and saturated fats increases serum levels of low-density lipoproteins (LDLs). These appear to promote arterial plaque. Evidence suggests, however, that other fats—high-density lipoproteins—protect against plaque formation, possibly by transporting cholesterol out of arterial lesions.

Diabetes mellitus
For reasons that aren't completely understood, many patients with diabetes mellitus—even those with well-controlled blood glucose levels—develop atherosclerosis.

Hypertension
Hypertension stresses the intima of blood vessels. This stress, combined with other factors, such as high LDL levels, contributes to atherosclerotic plaque formation.

Stress
Numerous studies show a connection between prolonged physical or emotional stress and atherosclerotic plaque formation.

Genetic factors
A person whose parents or siblings have CAD is at greater risk for atherosclerosis than a person whose relatives have healthy blood vessels. Additionally, atherosclerosis is more likely to develop at a relatively young age in a person with Type II familial hyperlipoproteinemia.

Smoking
A strong link exists between cigarette smoking and CAD, possibly because smoking increases the adhesive quality of platelets. Smoking also alters oxygenation: It increases serum carbon monoxide levels at the same time that it decreases the amount of oxygen needed to support healthy tissue. While the myocardium's demand for oxygen increases, the available supply decreases.

Sedentary life-style
In general, a person who exercises regularly is at lower risk for atherosclerosis than is an inactive person. One reason for this may be that exercise, particularly aerobic exercise, affects lipid metabolism and improves cardiac efficiency.

Obesity
The risk that atherosclerosis will develop rises for obese people, especially if they smoke or have hyperlipidemia. A contributing factor is a sedentary life-style.

Assessment findings

A patient suffering an acute MI usually has classic signs and symptoms. But keep in mind that some patients exhibit uncharacteristic signs and symptoms, whereas others have no signs and symptoms. In fact, about 25% of all MIs remain undiagnosed because the patient's complaints are atypical.

Patient complaint
The chief complaint of a patient with an acute MI is usually substernal chest pain or pressure. The patient may describe it as sharp or stabbing, a dull ache, or a squeezing sensation. He may also say that he feels as though he has indigestion. The pain may radiate down the arms (especially the left arm) or into the neck, jaw, or back. Other common symptoms include nausea, vomiting, severe indigestion, dizziness, and loss of consciousness. The patient may feel apprehensive and express a sense of impending doom.

Initially, you should ask the patient about his pain. After he describes the intensity and exact location, ask if anything alleviates or aggravates the pain. If the pain worsens with breathing, it may result from pericarditis. Also, find out when the pain began and whether a particular activity—such as exertion, eating, or extreme emotion—triggered it.

Unlike the pain of angina, the pain of an MI lasts for at least 20 minutes, may persist for several hours, and is unrelieved by rest. Typically, the pain remains unchanged, or decreases only slightly, after the patient takes sublingual nitroglycerin.

Physical examination
Typically, the patient will be diaphoretic and dyspneic. He may also reposition himself restlessly in an attempt to alleviate pain. Most likely, his skin will appear pale and feel cool and moist. He may also be dizzy and confused.

The patient may be hypotensive from diminished cardiac output. His heart rate typically will be regular and rapid (possibly between 100 and 110 beats/minute). It will slow as his pain and anxiety ease.

The patient's respiratory rate may be rapid because of anxiety or discomfort; however, tachypnea may also signal left ventricular failure. Typically, the patient's temperature will be normal at the initial examination, but expect it to rise to between 99° and 100° F (37.2° and 37.8° C) within 24 to 48 hours. His temperature may remain elevated for 3 to 8 days in response to myocardial tissue necrosis.

Auscultation findings
During auscultation, you'll usually hear normal first and second heart sounds (S_1 and S_2). If the patient has had an extensive infarction, you may hear a third sound (S_3). This sound indicates heart failure and necessitates prompt intervention to relieve fluid overload and increase cardiac contractility. If the patient has hypertension or CAD, a fourth heart sound (S_4) may develop. Called an atrial gallop, this sound reflects reduced ventricular compliance. If an S_4 develops, the patient will need long-term follow-up to guard against worsening hypertension or CAD, which could lead to heart failure in a damaged myocardium.

Additionally, you may hear a heart murmur resulting from stenotic or incompetent valves. A stenotic valve may trigger heart failure because the damaged myocardium may no longer generate the force needed to pump against the valve. An incompetent valve, on the other hand, may foster regurgitation of blood, further decreasing already impaired cardiac output.

If you detect a murmur, first determine whether it's a new or preexisting one. A new murmur—especially a systolic murmur—may indicate papillary muscle dysfunction from ischemia or infarction. It may also indicate that the infarction caused a ventricular septal defect. This calls for emergency intervention to stop the shunting of unoxygenated blood from the right to the left side of the heart. If you hear the murmur only when the patient has pain, ischemia is the most likely cause.

You may hear another sound—a pericardial friction rub resulting from inflammation. This sound, which mimics grating leather, may not develop until 24 to 72 hours after the MI. It's best heard from the fourth intercostal space to

Evolution of an acute MI

These three electrocardiogram strips show the characteristic changes of the phases of an acute myocardial infarction (MI).

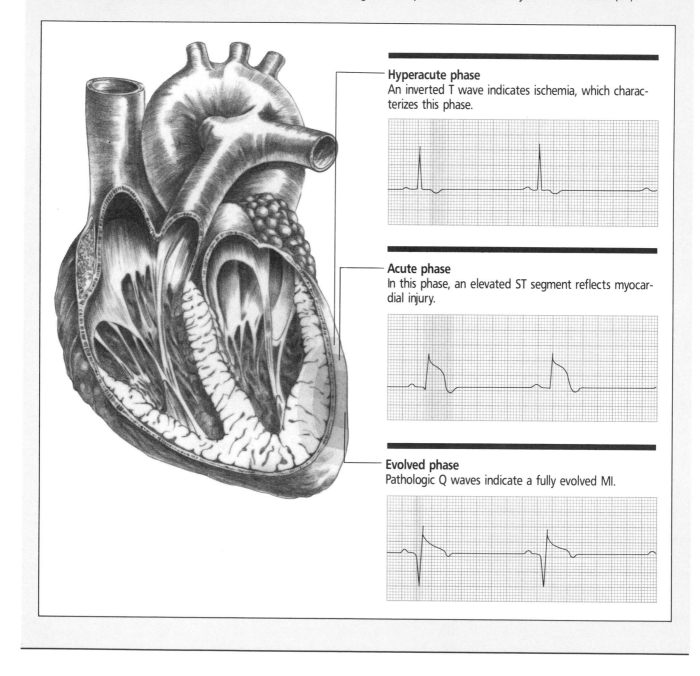

Hyperacute phase
An inverted T wave indicates ischemia, which characterizes this phase.

Acute phase
In this phase, an elevated ST segment reflects myocardial injury.

Evolved phase
Pathologic Q waves indicate a fully evolved MI.

ST-segment monitoring

The ST segment is a sensitive indicator of myocardial damage. Thus, by closely monitoring it, you can detect ischemia or injury before an infarction develops.

Keep in mind, though, that other conditions may alter the ST segment. They include electrolyte imbalances, oxygenation problems, heart chamber size, and various medications.

Normal ST segment
The ST segment, which represents the time between ventricular depolarization and repolarization, is normally an iso-electric line, as shown.

ST-segment depression
A deviation in the ST segment, such as a depression or an elevation, reflects a delay in conduction and depolarization. A depressed ST segment usually results from ischemia.

ST-segment elevation
An elevated ST segment usually results from myocardial injury. Prolonged ST-segment elevation may reflect pericarditis, reinfarction, ventricular aneurysm, or cardiac contusion.

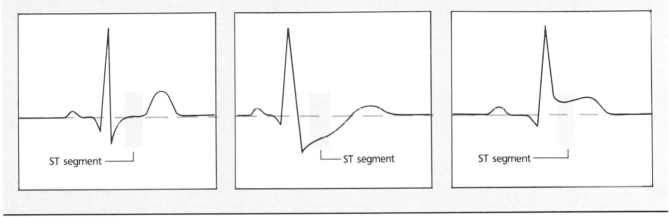

the right or left of the sternum. It often is only heard on deep inspiration. Once this sound exists, it may persist for 7 to 10 days.

After assessing the patient's heart sounds, you'll need to auscultate breath sounds. First, have the patient cough to clear his lungs. Then listen. If you hear crackles, notify the doctor. Such a finding may signal developing heart failure. Other signs of heart failure include increased heart and respiratory rates.

Characteristic ECG changes

The 12-lead ECG can be used to follow the development of an MI through three distinct phases: the hyperacute, the acute, and the evolved. During the hyperacute phase, myocardial tissue becomes ischemic. During the acute phase, myocardial injury develops. In the evolved stage, the MI occurs. Each of these phases produces its own characteristic ECG changes. Keep in mind that if the patient receives thrombolytic therapy, these ECG characteristics may be altered. (See *Evolution of an acute MI.*)

Be aware that many conditions can mimic an acute MI on a 12-lead ECG. These include diffuse myocardial disease, right or left ventricular hypertrophy, hypertrophic cardiomyopathy, anteroposterior hemiblock, Wolff-Parkinson-White syndrome, pancreatitis, pulmonary embolism, and subarachnoid hemorrhage. Also, use of a ventricular pacemaker may produce ECG changes that mimic those of an MI.

Locating myocardial damage

After you've noted one or more of the characteristic lead changes of an acute myocardial infarction, use this chart to identify the area of damage. Match the lead changes in the second column with the affected wall in the first column and the artery involved in the third column. Column four provides the reciprocal lead changes.

WALL AFFECTED	LEADS	ARTERY INVOLVED	RECIPROCAL CHANGES
Inferior (diaphragmatic)	II, III, aV$_F$	Right coronary artery	I, aV$_L$
Lateral	I, aV$_L$, V$_5$, V$_6$	Circumflex branch of left anterior descending (LAD) artery	V$_1$, V$_2$
Anterior	V$_2$, V$_3$, V$_4$	Left coronary artery	II, III, aV$_F$
Posterior	V$_1$, V$_2$, V$_3$	Right coronary artery, circumflex branch of left coronary artery	R wave greater than S wave; depressed ST segment; elevated T wave
Apical	V$_3$, V$_4$, V$_5$, V$_6$	LAD artery, right coronary artery	II, III, aV$_F$
Anterolateral	I, aV$_L$, V$_4$, V$_5$, V$_6$	LAD artery, circumflex branch of left coronary artery	II, III, aV$_F$
Anteroseptal	V$_1$, V$_2$, V$_3$	LAD artery	None

Hyperacute phase
During this initial phase of an MI, the ECG will initially show upright, peaked T waves and either elevated or depressed ST segments. When elevated ST segments appear, the T waves become inverted. For an ST segment to be considered depressed, it must remain at least 1 mm below the baseline for 0.08 second or more beyond the J point. (See *ST-segment monitoring,* page 101.)

During this phase, patients tend to develop ventricular arrhythmias or conduction defects.

Acute phase
As the patient's pain continues, the ischemic area of the myocardium sustains injury. In this phase, the leads monitoring the affected area will show elevated ST segments. In the leads opposite the affected area, known as the reciprocal leads, you'll see depressed ST segments.

Evolved phase
The appearance of pathologic Q waves signals the beginning of a fully evolved MI. These Q waves — which have a duration of 0.04 second and an amplitude of at least one-third the height of the QRS complex — occur when damaged tissue diverts the wave of depolarization from its normal path. Simultaneously, in the reciprocal leads, tall R waves may appear. This phase begins several hours after the onset of the MI and may continue for several weeks.

Permanent pathologic Q waves
As the patient's condition improves, first the ST segments and then the T waves return to normal. But the pathologic Q waves may remain as the only permanent change on his ECG.

In some cases, the ECG of a patient who has had an MI may never show pathologic Q waves. Traditionally, cardiologists have equated a lack of Q waves with a nontransmural MI,

Monitoring MI patients

Anterior wall MI

When monitoring a patient with an anterior wall myocardial infarction (MI)—who is at risk for heart block, ventricular arrhythmias, and ventricular septal defect—use lead V_1 because it shows the most comprehensive electrocardiogram changes. You can recognize changes in the ST segment that may indicate resolution of an MI or perhaps extension of infarction.

Lead V_1

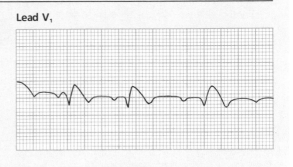

Lateral wall MI

To monitor a patient with a lateral wall MI, use lead V_6 or MCL_6. These leads give the best view of the lateral wall.

Lead V_6

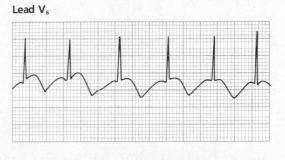

Inferior wall MI

Use lead II to monitor a patient with a recent inferior wall MI. This lead gives the best view of the inferior wall and thus the best view of extended. damage or reinfarction.

Lead II

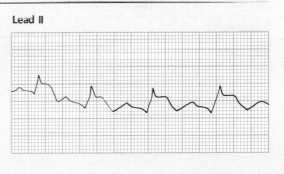

meaning that damage didn't extend through the entire cardiac wall. Studies now show, however, that the ECGs of some patients who suffer an acute transmural MI (an infarction that involves the full thickness of the cardiac wall) never exhibit pathologic Q waves. Conversely, some patients exhibit pathologic Q waves without having had a transmural MI.

Usually, pathologic Q waves indicate that the patient has had an MI in the past. If he denies having had one, he may have had an asymptomatic MI, sometimes called a silent MI.

Types of MIs

Usually, MIs are classified according to the portion of the myocardium they damage. The most common areas of damage include the anterior wall, the septal wall, the lateral wall, the

Recognizing an anterior wall MI

This 12-lead electrocardiogram shows the characteristics of an anterior wall myocardial infarction (MI). Note the absence of an R-wave progression in the precordial leads and the ST-segment elevation in leads V_2 and V_3. The reciprocal leads II, III, and aV_F show slight ST-segment depression.

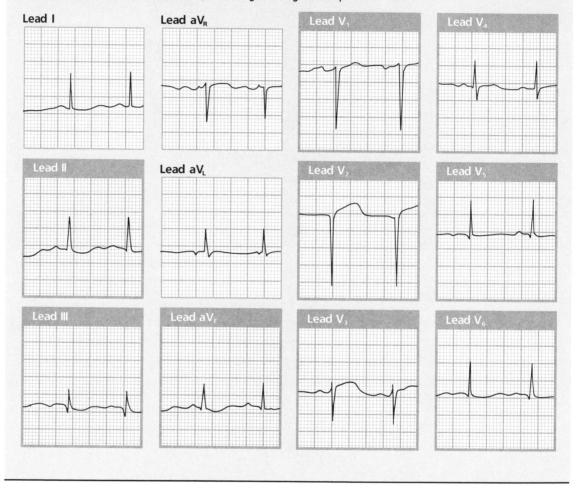

inferior wall, the right ventricle, and the posterior wall. Less common locations include the subendocardial, apical, and atrial areas.

You can determine the type (or location) of any MI by noting which leads show the characteristic ECG changes. (See *Locating myocardial damage,* page 102.)

Anterior wall MI
The main portion of the left coronary artery divides into the left anterior descending (LAD)

artery and the circumflex artery. The LAD artery supplies blood to the anterior portion of the ventricle. Thus, when an occlusion affects this artery, an anterior wall MI occurs. The LAD artery serves such an extensive portion of the heart that an occlusion commonly proves fatal.

Because the LAD artery supplies blood to the ventricular septum and portions of the right and left bundle-branch systems, complications of an anterior wall MI include varying de-

Recognizing an anteroseptal wall MI

This 12-lead electrocardiogram shows changes characteristic of an anterior wall myocardial infarction (MI) with septal involvement—commonly known as an anteroseptal wall MI. Note the poor R-wave progression in the precordial leads and the elevated ST segments and inverted T waves in leads V_1, V_2, and V_3. The reciprocal leads II, III, and aV_F show depressed ST segments and tall, peaked T waves.

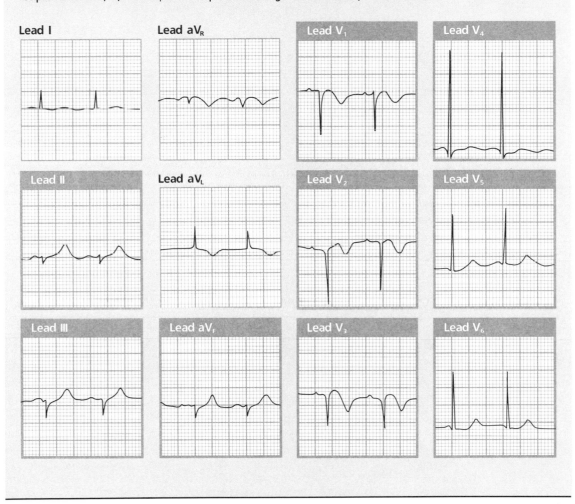

grees of heart block (usually bundle-branch blocks, Type II second-degree heart block, or complete heart block) and ventricular arrhythmias caused by left ventricular irritability. The patient with an anterior wall MI is also at risk for a ventricular septal defect, a ventricular aneurysm, a ventricular rupture, and left ventricular failure.

Characteristic ECG changes
With an anterior wall MI, the left ventricle doesn't depolarize normally. As a result, the precordial leads show poor R-wave progression along with ST-segment elevation and T-wave inversion. Because leads V_2, V_3, and V_4 lie directly over the left ventricle, they show the most obvious changes.

Leads II, III, and aV$_F$—which are reciprocal to leads V$_2$, V$_3$, and V$_4$—show strong R waves, depressed ST segments, and peaked T waves. Once you identify these changes, monitor the patient's ECG closely for any sign that the MI is extending into the septal or lateral wall. (See *Monitoring MI patients*, page 103, and *Recognizing an anterior wall MI*, page 104.)

Septal wall MI

Because the LAD artery also supplies blood to the ventricular septum, a septal wall MI commonly accompanies an anterior wall MI. The patient who suffers a septal wall MI is at increased risk for developing a ventricular septal defect.

Characteristic ECG changes

When a septal wall MI occurs, leads V$_1$ and V$_2$ detect the ECG changes. The R wave disappears—indicating defective septal depolarization—while the ST segment rises and the T wave inverts. These changes may occur alone, or they may accompany the changes associated with an anterior wall MI. (See *Recognizing an anteroseptal wall MI*, page 105.)

When you're caring for a patient who's at risk for a septal wall MI, monitor lead V$_1$ or MCL$_1$ to pick up these hallmark changes.

Lateral wall MI

The circumflex branch of the left main coronary artery furnishes blood to the lateral and posterior portions of the left ventricle. In about 40% of the population, it also supplies the left atrium, and in another 10% it supplies the atrioventricular (AV) node. So, when the circumflex artery occludes, an infarction occurs in the lateral wall of the left ventricle, typically causing such complications as premature ventricular contractions (PVCs) and varying degrees of heart block, such as first-degree or Type I second-degree heart block.

A lateral wall MI typically accompanies an anterior or inferior wall MI.

Characteristic ECG changes

Leads I, aV$_L$, V$_5$, and V$_6$ view the lateral wall. After a lateral wall MI, these leads usually show significant changes, such as elevated ST

segments, inverted T waves, and pathologic Q waves.

Reciprocal changes include ST-segment depression, tall T waves, and R-wave progression. When the anterior wall isn't affected, these changes appear in leads V$_1$ and V$_2$. When the inferior wall isn't affected, the reciprocal changes occur in leads II, III, and aV$_F$. (See *Recognizing an anterolateral wall MI*.)

Inferior wall MI

The right coronary artery normally supplies blood to the right ventricle, right atrium, sinus of Valsalva, a portion of the bundle-branch system, and—in many patients—the sinoatrial and AV nodes. When this artery becomes occluded, an inferior wall MI results. Because the inferior portion of the heart lies just above the diaphragm, an infarction in this area is commonly called a diaphragmatic MI.

When an inferior wall MI occurs, the patient is at risk for developing sinus bradycardia or sinus arrest. Other complications include first-degree or Type I second-degree heart block and PVCs. With extensive damage, the patient may suffer right ventricular failure.

An inferior wall MI may occur alone or in conjunction with a lateral wall MI or a right ventricular MI.

Characteristic ECG changes

Leads II, III, and aV$_F$, which provide the best views of the inferior portion of the heart, show the significant changes—elevated ST segments, inverted T waves, and pathologic Q waves. Reciprocal changes of ST-segment depression and tall T waves occur in leads I, aV$_L$ and, at times, V$_4$, V$_5$, and V$_6$. (See *Recognizing an inferior wall MI*, page 108.)

Right ventricular MI

A right ventricular MI usually follows occlusion of the right coronary artery. This MI rarely occurs alone. In fact, 40% of the patients who suffer an inferior wall MI also suffer a right ventricular MI. An infarction in the right ventricle can lead to right ventricular failure or right bundle-branch block.

Recognizing an anterolateral wall MI

This 12-lead electrocardiogram shows changes characteristic of an anterolateral myocardial infarction (MI). Note the pathologic Q waves, slight ST-segment elevation, and T-wave inversion in lead I. Also, examine the pathologic Q waves, the slightly elevated ST segments, and the inverted T waves in lead aV_L. These findings represent a lateral wall MI.

   Now examine the precordial leads. Observe the elevated ST segments and inverted T waves. These changes indicate damage involving the anterior wall.

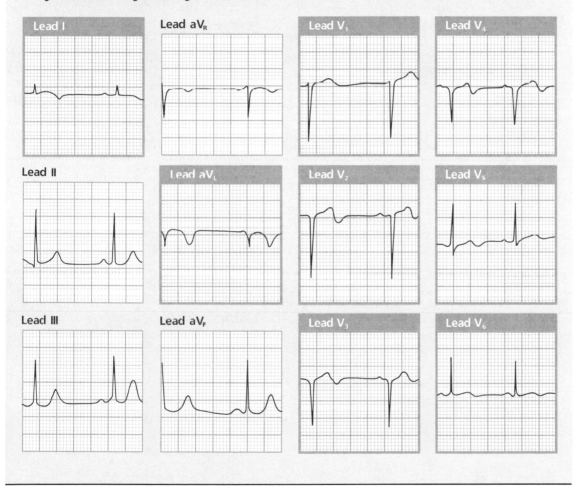

Characteristic ECG changes
With a right ventricular MI, the classic changes of ST-segment elevation, pathologic Q waves, and inverted T waves occur in the right precordial leads: V_2R, V_3R, V_4R, V_5R, and V_6R. To obtain right precordial lead readings, you must position the electrodes on the right side of the patient's chest, as follows:

• V_2R at the fourth intercostal space, right sternal border
• V_3R midway between V_2R and V_4R
• V_4R at the fifth intercostal space, right midclavicular line
• V_5R at the fifth intercostal space, right anterior axillary line
• V_6R at the fifth intercostal space, right midaxillary line.

Recognizing an inferior wall MI

This 12-lead electrocardiogram shows characteristic changes of an inferior wall myocardial infarction (MI). In leads II, III, and aV$_F$, note the T-wave inversion, ST-segment elevation, and pathologic Q waves. In leads I and aV$_L$, note the slight ST-segment depression, a reciprocal change.

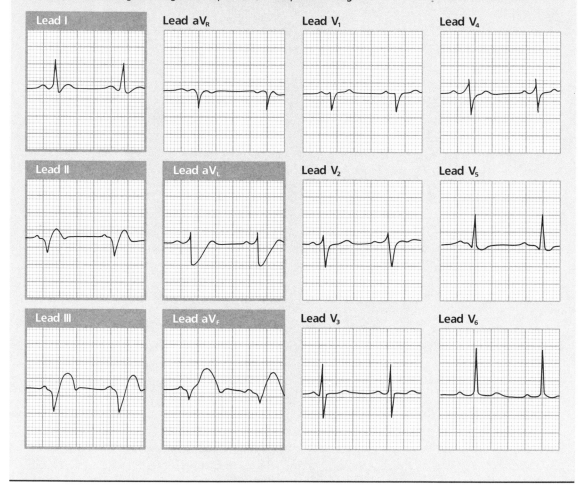

Without these leads, identifying a right ventricular MI is difficult. That's because ECG changes characteristic of a right ventricular MI are subtle and fleeting. If right precordial leads aren't available, observe leads II, III, and aV$_F$ for signs of an inferior wall MI. Also watch leads V$_1$, V$_2$, and V$_3$ for elevated ST segments.

If your patient has had a right ventricular MI, use lead V$_1$ to monitor him for further damage. (See *Recognizing a right ventricular MI*.)

Posterior wall MI
A posterior wall MI can result from an occluded right coronary artery or an occluded circumflex branch of the left coronary artery. These arteries feed the posterior portion of the right and left ventricles, so a blockage here commonly leads to ventricular failure.

Characteristic ECG changes
Patients suffering a posterior wall MI have only vague signs and symptoms, so your ECG find-

Recognizing a right ventricular MI

This 12-lead electrocardiogram shows the characteristics of a right ventricular myocardial infarction (MI): pathologic Q waves, ST-segment elevation, and inverted T waves in leads V_{3R}, V_{4R}, V_{5R}, and V_{6R}.

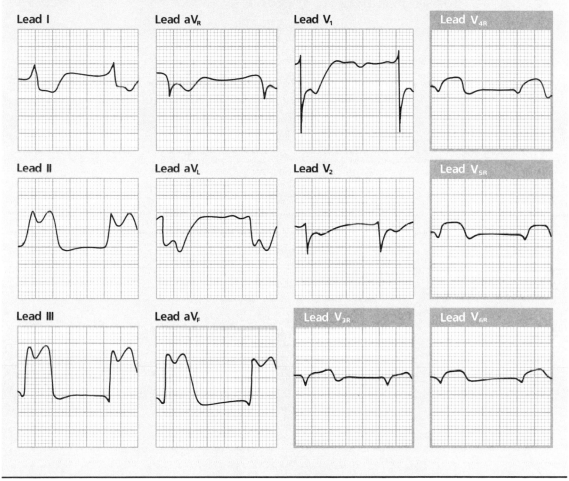

Lead I   Lead aV_R Lead V_1 Lead V_{4R}

Lead II   Lead aV_L Lead V_2 Lead V_{5R}

Lead III   Lead aV_F Lead V_{3R} Lead V_{6R}

ings are particularly important. Because none of the standard 12 leads directly views the posterior wall, you must depend on reciprocal changes in anterior leads — particularly leads V_1, V_2, and V_3 — to identify a posterior wall MI. These changes include R waves larger than S waves, depressed ST segments, and elevated T waves. When monitoring a patient who has had a posterior wall MI, use lead V_1 or MCL_1 for the best view. (See *Recognizing a posterior wall MI*, page 110, and *Direct view of a posterior wall MI*, page 111.)

Less common types of MIs
Your patient may also experience one of the less common types of MI, including subendocardial, apical, and atrial MIs.

Subendocardial MI
An infarction that damages only the surface of the inner ventricular lining is called a subendocardial MI. Because this type of MI usually doesn't produce pathologic Q waves, some clinicians call it a non–Q-wave (or nontransmural) MI.

Recognizing a posterior wall MI

This 12-lead electrocardiogram shows the characteristic changes of a posterior wall myocardial infarction (MI): tall R waves, depressed ST segments, and upright T waves in leads V_1, V_2, and V_3. These leads show you the reciprocal changes that occur when a posterior wall MI occurs.

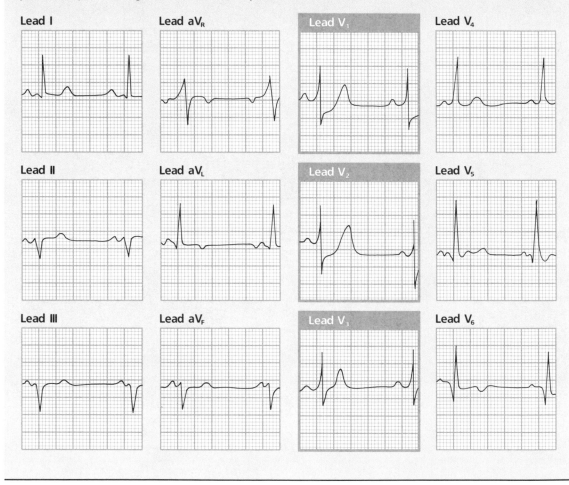

Lead I · Lead aV$_R$ · Lead V$_1$ · Lead V$_4$
Lead II · Lead aV$_L$ · Lead V$_2$ · Lead V$_5$
Lead III · Lead aV$_F$ · Lead V$_3$ · Lead V$_6$

Characteristic ECG changes
Patients suffering a posterior wall MI have only vague signs and symptoms, so your ECG findings are particularly important. Because none of the standard 12 leads directly views the posterior wall, you must depend on reciprocal changes in anterior leads — particularly leads V_1, V_2, and V_3 — to identify a posterior wall MI. These changes include R waves larger than S

Apical MI
An apical MI rarely occurs by itself. It usually is associated with an occlusion of the right coronary artery or of the LAD artery, which causes an inferior wall or anterior wall MI.

Characteristic ECG changes. To identify an apical MI, examine leads V_3, V_4, V_5, and V_6. You should observe a loss of R-wave progression, elevated ST segments, inverted T waves, and pathologic Q waves.

Atrial MI

An atrial MI also rarely occurs as an isolated event. It may accompany an infarction of the right or left ventricle.

Characteristic ECG changes. Typical ECG characteristics of an atrial MI include a prolonged PR interval and atrial arrhythmias.

Diagnostic studies

In many cases, additional studies are needed to confirm a diagnosis of MI and to evaluate the extent of myocardial damage. Other diagnostic tools include cardiac enzyme analysis, chest X-ray, echocardiography, magnetic resonance imaging (MRI), nuclear imaging, and cardiac catheterization.

Cardiac enzyme analysis

Enzymes—the protein catalysts that trigger many chemical reactions—reside in all cells. Changes in circulating enzyme levels may indicate an MI. Significant enzymes in diagnosing MI include creatine phosphokinase (CPK); lactate dehydrogenase (LDH); and aspartate aminotransferase (AST), formerly SGOT.

When an infarction damages myocardial tissue, these enzymes spill into the bloodstream. Elevated CPK levels are usually detected in the bloodstream 6 to 8 hours after an MI. CPK concentrations peak in about 24 hours and return to normal after about 4 days. Serum LDH levels begin to rise 24 to 48 hours after an infarction, peak in 3 to 6 days, and return to normal after 8 to 14 days. Finally, AST levels rise 8 to 12 hours after an infarction, peak in 18 to 36 hours, and return to normal in 3 to 4 days.

Keep in mind that LDH and AST exist in tissues outside the heart, so conditions other than an MI may cause these enzyme levels to rise.

Chest X-ray

Although not used specifically to diagnose an MI, a chest X-ray gives information about the heart's ability to pump blood by showing the

Direct view of a posterior wall MI

Normally, you'll identify a posterior wall myocardial infarction (MI) by recognizing reciprocal changes (depressed ST segments) in leads V_1, V_2, and V_3. But you can also identify this type of MI by creating leads that directly view the posterior wall. Place three additional electrodes on the patient's back to create leads V_7, V_8, and V_9. If your patient has a posterior wall MI, these leads will show the classic changes. All three leads will show elevated ST segments and inverted T waves; leads V_8 and V_9 will display pathologic Q waves.

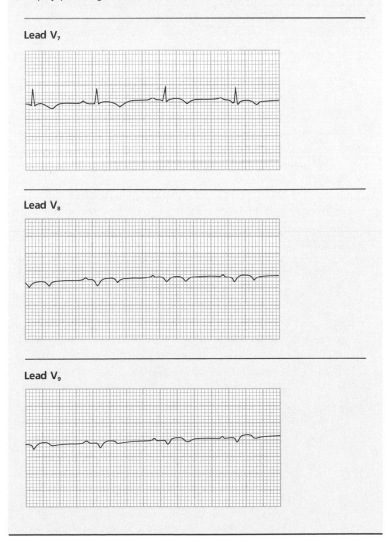

Lead V_7

Lead V_8

Lead V_9

heart's size. For example, cardiomegaly may point to pump impairment.

A chest X-ray can also detect pulmonary congestion—the first sign of heart failure. This may result from weakened heart contractions that permit blood to pool in the left ventricle, back up into the left atrium, and spill into the lungs. Typically, the X-ray film shows cloudiness or distended veins in the upper lung lobes.

If you're evaluating a patient's chest X-ray, be sure to compare a current film with a previous film. Also, keep in mind that cardiac abnormalities may not be apparent on a chest X-ray.

Echocardiography

Also called ultrasound imaging, echocardiography uses sound waves to produce a two-dimensional, cross-sectional view of the heart. By studying a patient's echocardiogram, you'll learn about the heart's size and shape. You can also assess movement in the myocardial walls and the spatial relationship of cardiac structures.

A variation of two-dimensional echocardiography, M-mode echocardiography produces a one-dimensional view of cardiac motion. By combining the two-dimensional and M-mode results, the doctor can assess damage to cardiac walls and valves.

Magnetic resonance imaging

Magnetic resonance imaging (MRI) produces pictures of soft structures. With MRI, the cardiologist can assess the heart chambers, ventricular mass, and the position of the heart and great vessels. Because MRI relies on magnetic fields—rather than radiation—to produce images, the study is considered safe during childhood and pregnancy. It's contraindicated, however, for patients with pacemakers or those with a surgically implanted metal part, such as a hip prosthesis or pin.

Nuclear imaging

Used to determine the exact size and site of an infarction and the motion of cardiac walls, nuclear imaging comprises a group of specific tests.

Technetium scanning

In this test, the doctor injects a small amount of a radioactive substance—technetium-99m stannous pyrophosphate—into the patient and waits while the dyelike substance accumulates in the damaged myocardial tissue. Here it creates a "hot spot" discernible by a special camera. The scan result shows the exact size and location of an infarction.

A hot spot usually becomes visible about 12 hours after an infarction and disappears within 1 week. Other conditions that may appear as a hot spot include ventricular aneurysm, heart or chest tumors, cardiac trauma, and myocardial damage resulting from defibrillation.

Thallium imaging

Similar to technetium scanning, thallium imaging also shows the site and extent of an MI. In this study, dyelike contrast material accumulates in healthy rather than damaged tissue, designating damaged areas (unmarked by dye) as "cold spots." These cold spots become visible within a few hours after an infarction.

Thallium imaging has several drawbacks. Damaged tissue can be difficult to visualize, and any area of decreased perfusion will show up as a cold spot. The resulting image may signify new damage, or it may show previous infarction or ischemia. Cold spots also appear in such conditions as sarcoidosis, myocardial fibrosis, cardiac contusion, and coronary spasm. Electrodes and breast implants will also appear as cold spots on a thallium scan.

Gated heart studies

Also called nuclear wall motion studies, gated heart studies are useful for assessing an MI's extent, judging overall cardiac function, and evaluating the effect of therapy. Combined with a stress test, the study helps determine the severity of CAD.

The test begins with an injection of blood or albumin that has been tagged with a radioactive substance. Over time, a camera records the movement of the tagged blood cells and, with it, the motion of the heart's walls.

First-pass studies record the movement of blood through the heart over one cardiac cycle. Additional studies, called multiple-gated acquisition (MUGA) scans, record heart motion over several hundred cycles. In MUGA scanning, the patient's ECG triggers the camera. By comparing end-diastolic and end-systolic counts of the tagged red blood cells, the doctor computes the patient's ejection fraction, which reflects ventricular strength.

Cardiac catheterization

An invasive test, cardiac catheterization provides valuable information about valvular function and ventricular motion. Combined with angiography, cardiac catheterization helps assess the patency of the coronary arteries.

The test involves inserting a catheter into the right or left side of the heart, or both. The doctor injects a radiopaque dye into the catheter, and the dye illuminates cardiac structures appearing on a monitor.

Catheterizing the heart's right side allows the doctor to study the tricuspid and pulmonary valves and right ventricular contractility. He can also diagnose intracardiac shunts and pulmonary hypertension, determine cardiac output, and measure electrical conduction.

By inserting the catheter into the heart's left side, the doctor can assess the mitral and aortic valves and left ventricular contractility.

If the doctor will also perform angiography, he'll advance the catheter past the aortic valve into the coronary ostia and then inject dye. This dye then circulates to reveal coronary arteries that remain patent, previous bypass graft sites, and arterial spasms. The dye also permits the doctor to measure the amount of collateral circulation that develops after an MI.

Treatment

The goal of MI treatment is to preserve as much myocardial tissue as possible by increasing oxygen supply to the myocardium and decreasing the cardiac work load. Besides rest, pain relief, and supplemental oxygen, various medications and procedures are used to accomplish this.

Medications

Some medications dilate the coronary arteries, which increases the volume of oxygen reaching myocardial tissue. Other medications reduce myocardial demand for oxygen by slowing the heart rate, decreasing the force of contractions, easing the preload, or decreasing the afterload. Still other medications relieve pain, which is an initial treatment goal.

Nitroglycerin, morphine sulfate, beta blockers, and calcium channel blockers are commonly prescribed after an MI.

Nitroglycerin

A key drug in cardiotherapy, nitroglycerin may be given I.V. because sublingual administration is usually ineffective after an MI. Given I.V., nitroglycerin relieves pain and dilates blood vessels (both coronary arteries) to improve myocardial and peripheral circulation. Such systemic vasodilation reduces afterload, which, in turn, decreases the heart's work load.

Administer I.V. nitroglycerin cautiously. Always mix the drug in a glass bottle because the medication adheres to plastic. Also check to see if your institution uses special I.V. tubing for administering nitroglycerin. Be sure to use an infusion pump so that you can titrate the drug according to the patient's blood pressure and pain level. During administration, closely monitor the patient's vital signs, and remain alert for signs of hypotension, which can result from vasodilation.

Morphine sulfate

When nitroglycerin fails to relieve pain, or when the dose is being titrated, I.V. morphine sulfate may be ordered. This drug effectively relieves pain as it promotes slight vasodilation to decrease myocardial work load.

Beta blockers

Also serving to reduce myocardial work load, beta blockers inhibit catecholamine stimulation of beta$_1$- and beta$_2$-adrenergic receptors. This slows the heart rate and decreases contractility, which, in turn, decreases cardiac work load and eases oxygen demand.

Thrombolytic therapy: Indications and contraindications

To receive a thrombolytic agent, a patient must have:
• symptoms consistent with an acute myocardial infarction (MI)
• chest pain unrelieved by nitroglycerin and of fewer than 6 hours' duration
• electrocardiogram patterns characteristic of an acute MI.

Factors that preclude thrombolytic therapy include:
• recent major surgery, organ biopsy, or puncture of a major blood vessel
• recent delivery of a baby
• recent trauma
• recent cardiopulmonary resuscitation
• severe, uncontrolled hypertension
• cerebrovascular accident
• pregnancy
• bleeding disorders
• internal hemorrhage
• intracranial neoplasm
• atrioventricular malformation.

Calcium channel blockers

Calcium channel blockers inhibit the flow of calcium into cells. As a result, vascular smooth muscle relaxes, and the coronary arteries and peripheral vessels dilate. This increases oxygen flow to the myocardium and reduces myocardial work load.

Thrombolytic therapy

Increasingly used for acute MIs, thrombolytic therapy involves dissolving a thrombus with a drug injected either I.V. or directly into the affected coronary artery during coronary angiography. Common thrombolytic agents include streptokinase, urokinase, tissue plasminogen activator (t-PA or alteplase), and anistreplase. Although thrombolytic therapy may effectively promote reperfusion, remember that the artery can still reocclude. (See *Thrombolytic therapy: Indications and contraindications.*)

Complications. Minor complications can result from thrombolytic therapy. They include bleeding from the gums or the puncture site. To minimize the risk of bleeding, take steps to protect the patient. For example, advise him to use a soft toothbrush. If bleeding occurs at the puncture site, you can usually control it with direct pressure.

If serious bleeding occurs — for example, if neurologic changes point to intracranial bleeding, or if vital signs change and falling hematocrit levels suggest internal bleeding — stop the infusion immediately, and notify the doctor.

Monitoring the patient. Watch the patient's ECG monitor to determine the effectiveness of therapy. Suppose, for example, that the patient's ECG initially showed elevated ST segments. If the ST segment returns to baseline after thrombolytic therapy, you can conclude that the thrombus dissolved. Other signs of reperfusion include an accelerated idioventricular rhythm, pain relief, and an early peak in serum CPK levels.

Other medications

The patient recovering from an MI may receive other drugs to decrease ventricular automaticity and help prevent arrhythmias. Although I.V. lidocaine remains the drug of choice, other effective agents include procainamide and bretylium. The patient also may receive medications to treat complications — for example, atropine for a conduction disorder, inotropic agents to relieve severe heart failure by boosting the heart's pumping action, or a vasodilator to ease cardiac work load.

Intra-aortic balloon pump

Depending on the patient's age, the blood vessel involved, the patient's response to treatment, and any complications, the doctor may decide to insert an intra-aortic balloon pump (IABP). The IABP relieves chest pain and decreases the infarction's size by promoting blood flow to the myocardium and increasing collateral circulation. The device also improves peripheral circulation and decreases the heart's work load.

Other treatments

Another method of restoring patency to an occluded coronary vessel is percutaneous transluminal coronary angioplasty (PTCA). Performed during cardiac catheterization, PTCA involves inserting a balloon-tipped catheter into the stenotic coronary artery. The doctor then inflates the balloon, which dilates the vessel.

Or the patient may require a coronary artery bypass graft to restore myocardial circulation. This surgical procedure involves removing a vein—usually a portion of the saphenous vein—and attaching it to the coronary artery in such a way that it bypasses the obstruction.

Other ways of improving blood flow include surgically placing a stent in the occluded artery or performing a coronary atherectomy. In the latter procedure, which is performed with coronary angiography, the doctor uses a fine scalpel to scrape plaque from inside an artery.

Cardiac rehabilitation

After the patient recovers sufficiently, he may enter a cardiac rehabilitation program. Such a program involves the patient in systematic and structured exercise while ensuring his safety by cardiac monitoring. As his condition improves, the patient may begin exercising at home. The patient's increased activity level not only improves his cardiovascular health but also boosts his self-esteem.

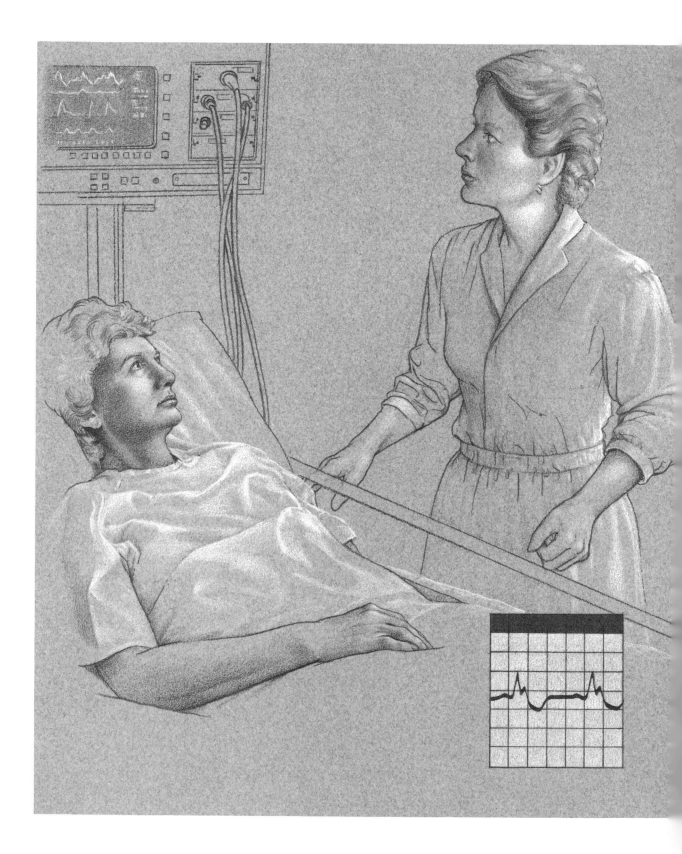

9

CHAPTER

Heart blocks

Also called an interventricular conduction block, a heart block refers to impaired impulse conduction in one or more of the fascicles distal to the bundle of His—the right bundle branch, the left bundle branch, the left anterior fascicle, or the left posterior fascicle. Any of these conduction pathways may become completely or partially blocked, particularly in a patient who has heart disease.

Identifying a heart block on a 12-lead electrocardiogram (ECG) requires considerable knowledge and skill. This chapter will provide you with the information and help you attain the necessary skills to recognize the various types of heart blocks. These include right bundle-branch block (RBBB), left bundle-branch block (LBBB), left anterior hemiblock (LAHB), and left posterior hemiblock (LPHB), as well as bifascicular and trifascicular blocks.

The chapter begins with a brief review of normal ventricular activation and an overview of the causes of heart blocks. Next comes a discussion of assessment findings and characteristic ECG changes for all types of heart blocks. Then you'll find sections that provide specific information on the various types of heart blocks. The last section of the chapter covers treatment for heart blocks.

Causes

As you know, electrical impulses normally travel from the atrioventricular (AV) node to the bundle of His. Then they move synchronously through the right bundle branch and left bundle branch and its fascicles, and finally on to the Purkinje network, where ventricular activation takes place. The shorter, left main portion of the left bundle branch divides into the left anterior fascicle and the left posterior fascicle. Consequently, the distal conduction system is trifascicular, with impulses traveling along three routes after leaving the bundle of His.

Normally, the interventricular septum is activated first, with the impulse traveling faster down the left bundle branch than the right bundle branch. Thus, the interventricular septum is activated from left to right. Once the septum is activated, both ventricles are depolarized at the same time from the endocardial to the epicardial surface. Because the right ventricular wall is thinner than the left, activation of the right ventricle is completed first. The left ventricle is activated from the apex to base. (See *Normal ventricular activation.*)

An impulse may be blocked (a complete heart block) or delayed (an incomplete heart block) at any of the three fascicles. Simultaneous blockage in more than one fascicle produces a bifascicular or trifascicular block, and blockage at the bundle of His causes a complete heart block. (See *Abnormal ventricular activation,* pages 120 and 121.)

Typically, the right bundle branch and the left anterior fascicle are more prone to blockage than the left posterior fascicle or the bundle of His. The right bundle branch is vulnera-

ble because it's long and thin and supplied solely by the left anterior descending coronary artery. The left anterior fascicle is susceptible because it lies in the turbulent area of the left ventricle's outflow tract and has only one blood supply—again the left anterior descending coronary artery. In most people, the left anterior descending coronary artery and the right coronary artery branches supply blood to the left posterior fascicle. Given this dual blood supply, when a block of the left posterior fascicle does occur, it may indicate a serious cardiac disease. The bundle of His also receives blood from both the left anterior descending coronary artery and the right coronary artery branches.

Both temporary and permanent heart blocks may be associated with acute myocardial infarction (MI). An acute MI, in fact, is the primary cause of heart blocks. Other causes include atherosclerosis, valvular disease, ventricular hypertrophy, infective cardiac disease, primary heart disease, congenital abnormalities, and cardiac drugs that alter the refractory period of interventricular conduction.

Assessment findings

Most patients with bundle-branch blocks are asymptomatic, unless they also have other cardiac problems. Thus, with most patients the only way to identify a block is to perform and interpret an ECG.

When you assess a patient who has a bundle-branch block, keep in mind that a preexisting block isn't as serious as a new one caused by an acute condition, such as an MI. Also keep in mind that an acute MI may block more than one fascicle. What's more, you'll need to closely monitor any patient with a history of LBBB because two fascicles are already blocked. This condition will only be evident on an ECG; it produces no signs and symptoms.

(Text continues on page 122.)

Normal ventricular activation

This illustration shows the normal sequence of electrical stimulation in the ventricles. First, an electrical impulse activates the interventricular septum from left to right (1). Then, the impulse travels down the right bundle branch, the left bundle branch, and the left anterior and left posterior fascicles, activating the right and left ventricles (2).

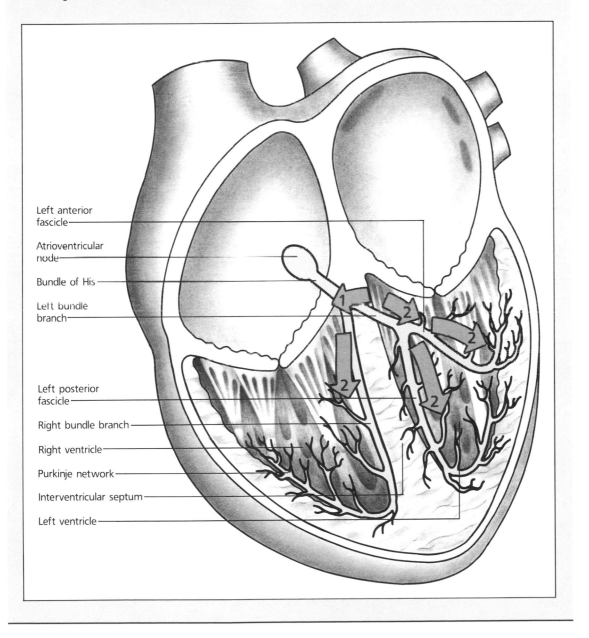

Left anterior fascicle

Atrioventricular node

Bundle of His

Left bundle branch

Left posterior fascicle

Right bundle branch

Right ventricle

Purkinje network

Interventricular septum

Left ventricle

PATHOPHYSIOLOGY

Abnormal ventricular activation

The following illustrations show the abnormal ventricular activation that occurs with right bundle-branch block (RBBB), left bundle-branch block (LBBB), left anterior hemiblock (LAHB), and left posterior hemiblock (LPHB).

Right bundle-branch block

In RBBB, the initial impulse activates the interventricular septum from left to right, just as in normal activation (1). Next, the left bundle branch activates the left ventricle (2). The impulse then crosses the interventricular septum to activate the right ventricle (3).

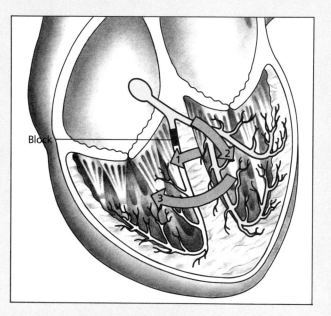

Left bundle-branch block

In LBBB, the impulse first travels down the right bundle branch (1). Then the impulse activates the interventricular septum from right to left, just the opposite of normal activation (2). Finally, the impulse activates the left ventricle (3).

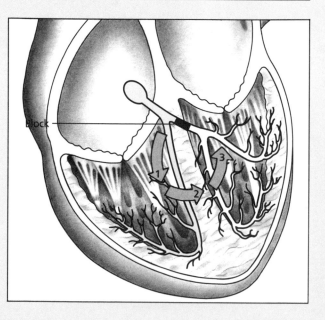

Left anterior hemiblock

In LAHB, the left ventricle is activated by the left posterior fascicle only (1). This causes the impulse to be aimed downward and to the right initially. After it reaches the Purkinje network, the impulse activates the anterior, lateral, and upper left ventricular walls (2).

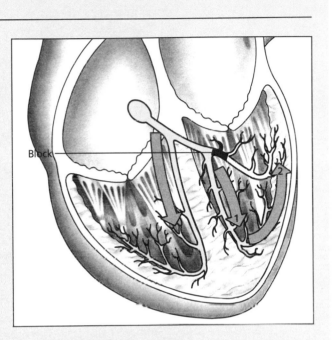

Left posterior hemiblock

In LPHB, the left anterior fascicle depolarizes the anterolateral wall of the left ventricle; at the same time, the right ventricle will be depolarized by the right bundle branch (1). After the impulse reaches the Purkinje network, it activates the inferoposterior wall of the left ventricle (2).

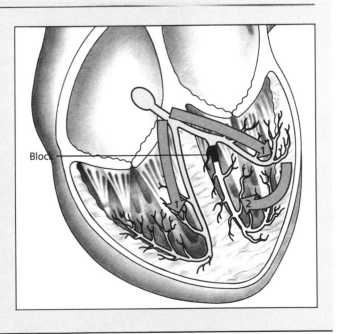

Characteristic ECG changes

A bundle-branch block causes asynchronous ventricular activation, which is reflected on the ECG. Depending on the particular type of block, the shape of the QRS complex will vary. To help understand these variations, take a few minutes now to review the normal shape of the QRS complex in two key leads: V_1 and V_6.

The positive electrode in V_1 is located over the fourth intercostal space at the right sternal border; the positive electrode in V_6, over the fifth intercostal space on the midaxillary line. So V_1 is directly to the right of the heart, and V_6, directly to the left.

Uppercase and lowercase letters distinguish between the relative sizes of the QRS complex components. For example, when the ventricular impulse that depolarizes the interventricular septum from left to right moves toward the positive electrode of V_1, it causes a small positive deflection (r wave). As the impulse moves toward the right ventricular epicardium, it also travels toward the positive pole of V_1, enhancing the R wave. Finally, the impulse moves away from the positive pole of V_1, causing a negative deflection (S wave). The S wave is large because the left ventricular wall is the thickest part of the heart.

By contrast, the impulse that depolarizes the interventricular septum from left to right travels away from the positive electrode of V_6. This causes a small negative deflection (q wave). As the impulse moves toward the right ventricle, it travels away from the positive pole of V_6, causing a more negative deflection (Q wave). Last, when the thick, left ventricular wall is depolarized, the impulse moves toward V_6, creating a large R wave.

Besides the distinctive shape of the QRS complex, heart blocks produce other ECG changes. With a complete RBBB or LBBB, for example, you'll note that the QRS complex has a longer duration. This, of course, reflects the delayed ventricular conduction. With a hemiblock, the QRS complex duration is normal because only part of the left bundle branch is blocked. The other fascicle can still depolarize part of the left ventricle.

The abnormal repolarization caused by a block will produce T-wave inversion in the lead located over the affected ventricle. In a patient with RBBB, for example, the T-wave inversion will appear in lead V_1; in a patient with LBBB, it will appear in V_6. A T wave with the same deflection as the terminal part of the QRS complex may signal additional heart disease and is called a primary change.

Because hemiblocks alter repolarization, they usually cause T-wave inversion as well.

Types of heart blocks

The different types of heart blocks—RBBB, LBBB, LAHB, LPHB, bifascicular block, and tri-fascicular block—stem from different causes and have different implications for the patient. And, of course, each type produces distinctive changes on a 12-lead ECG.

Right bundle-branch block

When an RBBB occurs, the impulse still activates the interventricular septum from left to right. But then the impulse activates the left ventricle before activating the right ventricle. (See *Recognizing RBBB*.)

Causes
An RBBB is usually associated with an anterior wall MI. If the block occurs within 3 days of an MI, the patient has twice the risk of progressing to complete heart block as would a patient with LBBB. When an RBBB occurs after 3 days, a complete AV block is less likely to develop.

Other common causes of an RBBB include coronary artery disease (CAD) and right ventricular hypertrophy. An RBBB may also result from pulmonary embolism, hypertension, rheumatic disease, cardiomyopathy, trauma, tumors, congenital lesions, and surgical correction of a ventricular-septal defect or tetralogy of Fallot. In some patients, an RBBB occurs without car-

Recognizing RBBB

This 12-lead electrocardiogram shows the characteristic changes of right bundle-branch block (RBBB). All leads have a prolonged QRS complex. In lead V_1, note the rsR' pattern and T-wave inversion. In lead V_6, note the widened S wave and the upright T wave.

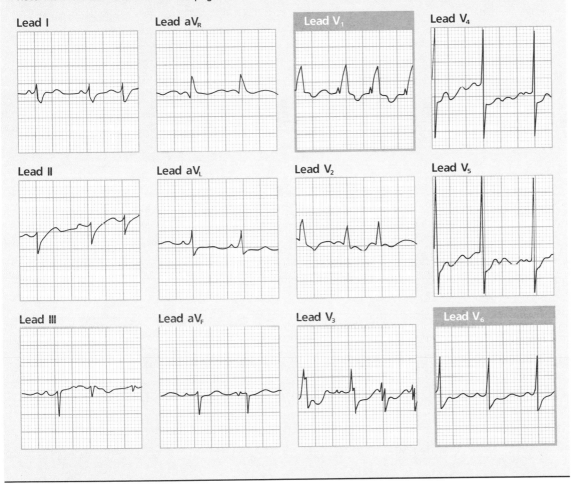

diac disease. An RBBB can develop as the heart rate increases (called rate-related RBBB).

Characteristic ECG changes
When right ventricular conduction is altered, distinctive changes occur on the patient's ECG. When the interventricular septum is initially activated from left to right by the left bundle branch, you'll see a small r wave in lead V_1 and a small q wave in lead V_6. Next, the left bundle branch activates the left ventricle, so

the impulse moves away from the positive pole of V_1, producing an S wave, and toward the positive pole of V_6, producing an R wave. The impulse then crosses the interventricular septum to activate the right ventricle, moving toward V_1 and producing another positive R wave, known as R prime (R'), and moving away from V_6 and producing an S wave.

Thus, in lead V_1 the QRS complex will have an rsR' pattern; in lead V_6, a qRS pattern. Although the left ventricle is activated before the right ventricle (the opposite of the normal sequence), the initial impulse still activates each ventricle in a normal way—from left to right.

In lead V_1, you'll see:
• an rSR′ pattern
• a prolonged QRS complex (exceeding 0.12 second)
• T-wave inversion.

In lead V_6, you'll see:
• a widened S wave
• a prolonged QRS complex (exceeding 0.12 second)
• an upright T wave.

Left bundle-branch block

In an LBBB, conduction through the left ventricle is impaired. A block may be located on the main bundle, or blocks may be located on both the anterior and posterior fascicles.

With an LBBB, ventricular activation occurs in this order: First, the right ventricle is activated by the right bundle branch. Then the interventricular septum is activated abnormally in a right-to-left direction. And, finally, the left ventricle is activated.

Causes
When LBBB is discovered on a routine ECG, the patient may have hypertensive ischemic disease, primary heart disease, or no serious heart disease at all.

Severe CAD, hypertensive cardiovascular disease, and valvular disease represent the most common causes of LBBB. Cardiomyopathy, Lev's disease, Lenegre's disease, rheumatic disease, and congenital lesions may also produce LBBB.

Characteristic ECG changes
Altered left ventricular activation produces characteristic changes on the patient's ECG.

In lead V_1, you'll see:
• a QS or rS pattern
• a prolonged QRS complex (exceeding 0.12 second).

In lead V_6, you'll see:
• an absent septal q wave. The right bundle branch activates the interventricular septum

from right to left, so the impulse moves toward the V_6 electrode, resulting in an initial positive deflection on the ECG. This characteristic is diagnostic.
• a tall, notched R wave. The right ventricle is activated after the interventricular septum. The initial positive R wave curves slightly downward because the impulse moves away from the V_6 electrode and toward the right ventricle. This curve or notch may look like a slurring of the R wave. The impulse then crosses back toward the left ventricle, activating it. The terminal part of the complex (the R wave) is positive because activation is toward lead V_6.
• a prolonged QRS complex. The duration may be as long as 0.16 second because the ventricles are activated sequentially, not simultaneously.
• T-wave inversion. The T wave will have a negative deflection because the terminal part of the QRS complex is positive. (See *Recognizing LBBB*.)

Anterior wall MI
Sometimes, identifying an associated MI can be difficult. That's because LBBB creates a unfamiliar ECG pattern that can hide the MI characteristics. An anterior wall MI is especially difficult to diagnose because one of its key characteristics is the Q wave in leads V_1 and V_2. And in an LBBB, the normal r wave in V_1 may be replaced by a QS pattern. So to detect an anterior wall MI in a patient with an LBBB, look for Q waves in leads I, aV_L, and V_6. If they're present, the patient probably has an anterior wall MI. You can also look for the ST-segment changes characteristic of MI in these same leads. If possible, compare one of the patient's previous ECGs with the current one.

Left anterior hemiblock

A blockage of the left anterior fascicle causes the left ventricle to be activated by the left posterior fascicle only. Impulses from this fascicle depolarize the inferior and posterior walls of the left ventricle. The right ventricle is depolarized by the right bundle branch at the same time. This causes the impulse to be aimed

Recognizing LBBB

This 12-lead electrocardiogram shows characteristic changes of a left bundle-branch block (LBBB). All leads have prolonged QRS complexes. In lead V_1, note the QS pattern. In lead V_6, note the notched R wave and the T-wave inversion.

The elevated ST segments and upright T waves in leads V_1 through V_4 are also common in LBBB.

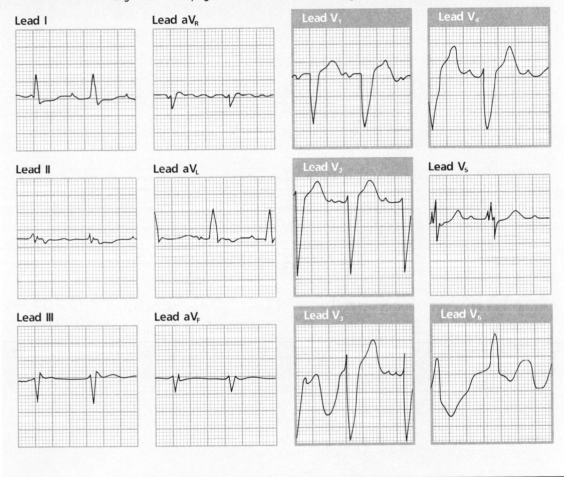

downward and to the right at first. After reaching the Purkinje network, the impulse activates the anterior, lateral, and upper left ventricular walls.

Causes

An LAHB can occur with an inferior wall MI, but it's more common with an acute anterior wall MI. An LAHB can also result from CAD, hypertension, cardiomyopathies, and aortic valve disease. LAHB is also associated with abdominal distention, obesity, and pregnancy. In these cases, the LAHB is temporary—most likely caused by left axis deviation rather than actual bundle blockage. Rarely, patients with no history of heart disease develop LAHB.

Characteristic ECG changes

LAHB causes distinctive changes on the patient's ECG.

Recognizing LAHB

This 12-lead electrocardiogram shows the characteristic changes of a left anterior hemiblock (LAHB). In leads II, III, and aV$_F$, note the rS pattern. In leads I and aV$_L$, note the qR pattern.

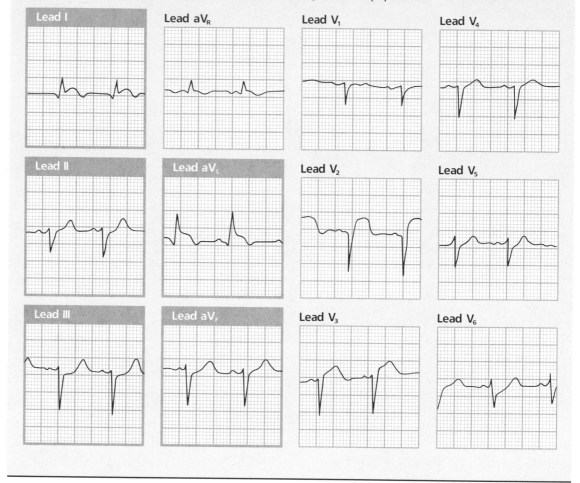

In leads II, III, and aV$_F$, you'll see an rS pattern. At first, the impulse moves swiftly through the left posterior fascicle, activating the inferior and posterior left ventricular walls, which are monitored by leads II, III, and aV$_F$. The initial deflection is positive (an r wave) because the impulse moves toward the positive poles first. But it goes only a short distance, so the r wave is small. The impulse then reaches the Purkinje network, activating the anterior and lateral left ventricular walls. Because the impulse travels a long distance away from the positive poles of leads II, III, and aV$_F$, a large terminal S wave appears.

In leads I and aV$_L$, you'll see a qR pattern. The inferior and posterior left ventricular walls, which are activated by the left posterior fascicle, are located away from the positive poles of leads I and aV$_L$. So the initial deflection is a small q wave. When the impulse travels through the Purkinje network and activates the anterior and lateral walls, it's moving toward the positive poles of leads I and aV$_L$. Thus, you'll see a large terminal R wave.

Recognizing LPHB

This 12-lead electrocardiogram shows the characteristic changes of a left posterior hemiblock (LPHB). In leads I and aV_L, note the rS pattern. In leads II, III, and aV_F, note the qR pattern.

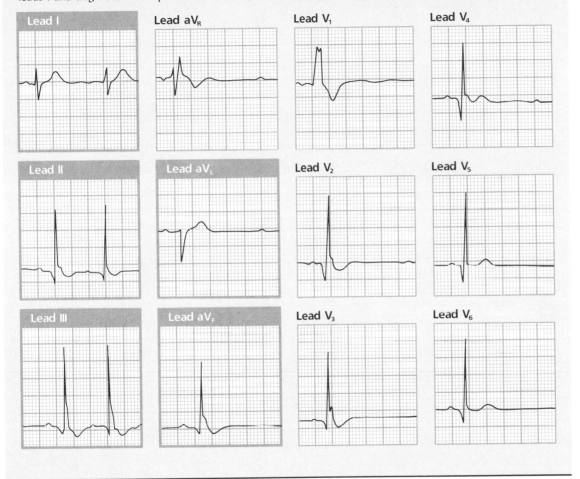

In all leads, you'll see a normal QRS complex duration. Because the impulse stays within the rapid conduction system, ventricular activation usually takes place within normal limits. However, the duration of the QRS complex will be slightly longer than the patient's baseline QRS complex duration.

With an LAHB, you may also note a left axis deviation. Some experts say the axis must be at least −45 degrees; others say that it only needs to be greater than −30 degrees. (See *Recognizing LAHB*.)

Inferior wall MI

One difficulty in assessing for LAHB is that it mimics other disorders, especially an inferior wall MI. The q wave is an important characteristic in diagnosing inferior wall damage. But in LAHB, the original deflection in leads II, III, and aV_F is an r wave, which helps prevent q wave formation. LAHB can also be mistaken for left ventricular hypertrophy.

Monitoring heart blocks

When your patient is on a bedside monitor, you need to select the single lead that best shows the type of block you're looking for.

Right bundle-branch block

Lead V_1 (or MCL_1) is best for identifying right bundle-branch block because this lead sits over the right ventricle, where the blockage occurs. Look for the pattern of rSR′ with secondary T-wave inversion and for a QRS complex duration greater than 0.12 second, as shown.

Lead V_1

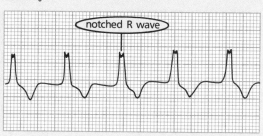

Left bundle-branch block

Lead V_6 (or MCL_6) is best for identifying left bundle-branch block. With this block, the electrical force is directed toward the left ventricle, producing a notched R wave in V_6 with T-wave inversion. Note the absence of a septal q wave.

Lead V_6

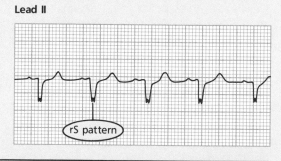

Left anterior hemiblock

Lead II is best for detecting left anterior hemiblock. With this abnormality, the QRS complex is negative in this lead and will have an rS pattern. Normally in this lead, the QRS complex is positive.

Lead II

Left posterior hemiblock

Lead I is best for monitoring a left posterior hemiblock. The electrical force is first deflected left and superiorly, toward the positive electrode of lead I, producing an r wave. Then the impulse is directed to the right and inferiorly, away from the positive electrode of lead I, producing an S wave. The QRS complex may or may not be prolonged.

Lead I

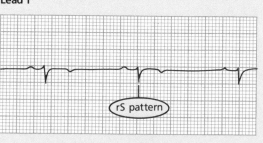

Left posterior hemiblock

With this type of block, the left anterior fascicle depolarizes the anterior and lateral walls of the left ventricle first. The right ventricle is depolarized by the right bundle branch at the same time. The impulse then crosses the Purkinje network and activates the inferior and posterior walls of the left ventricle. The impulse first moves to the left and anteriorly, then to the right and inferiorly.

Causes
This blockage usually occurs with an acute MI or ischemia or with CAD. Because patients with an acute MI and LPHB usually also have RBBB, the prognosis is poor. Other causes include aging, conduction system sclerosis, myocarditis, and hyperkalemia.

Characteristic ECG changes
LPHB causes characteristic changes on the patient's ECG.

In leads I and aV_L, you'll see an rS pattern. The initial impulse moves rapidly toward these leads, making the initial QRS complex deflection a small r wave. When the impulse moves to the right and inferiorly, it moves away from the positive poles of leads I and aV_L, creating a large terminal S wave.

In leads II, III, and aV_F, you'll see a qR pattern. Because the impulse first moves swiftly toward the anterior and lateral left ventricular walls and away from the positive poles of these leads, it creates a small q wave. Then, the impulse moves toward the inferior and posterior walls, creating a large terminal R wave in the inferior leads.

With LPHB, you'll also note a right axis deviation of +120 degrees. (See *Recognizing LPHB*, page 127, and *Monitoring heart blocks*.)

Right ventricular hypertrophy
In the limb leads, right ventricular hypertrophy causes the same ECG changes as LPHB.

Bifascicular block

Blockage of the RBBB and one of the left fascicles is known as bifascicular block. The most common combination is RBBB and LAHB because the roots of the right bundle branch and the left anterior fascicle are close together, and because these bundles receive blood from the same artery. A combination of RBBB and LPHB, less common but more serious, suggests more diffuse heart disease.

With RBBB and LAHB, the left posterior fascicle activates the left ventricle. The impulse first depolarizes the inferior and posterior left ventricular walls. Next, it activates the Purkinje network, depolarizing the anterior, lateral, and upper walls of the left ventricle. Finally, it reaches the right ventricle via the interventricular septum.

With RBBB and LPHB, the left anterior fascicle activates the left ventricle, first depolarizing the anterior, lateral, and upper walls. The impulse then travels through the Purkinje network to depolarize the inferior and posterior left ventricular walls. Finally, it activates the right ventricle through the interventricular septum.

A new bifascicular block occurring along with an acute MI can signal widespread necrosis of the ventricular myocardium and interventricular septum.

Causes
Hypertension and CAD are two common causes of RBBB and LAHB. Causes of RBBB and LPHB include CAD and anterior and inferior wall MIs with septal involvement.

Characteristic ECG changes
With RBBB and LAHB, you'll see a combination of the characteristics that signify the two abnormalities:
• in lead V_1, an rSR' pattern
• in lead V_6, a qRs pattern
• in leads II, III, and aV_F, an rS pattern
• in leads I and aV_L, a qR pattern
• left axis deviation.
(See *Recognizing bifascicular block: RBBB and LAHB*, page 130.)

With RBBB and LPHB, you'll see a combina-

Recognizing bifascicular block: RBBB and LAHB

This 12-lead electrocardiogram shows characteristic changes of a bifascicular block consisting of right bundle-branch block (RBBB) and left anterior hemiblock (LAHB). The rSR' pattern in lead V_1 and the qRs pattern in lead V_6 indicate RBBB. The rS pattern in leads II, III, and aV_F and the qR pattern in leads I and aV_L indicate LAHB.

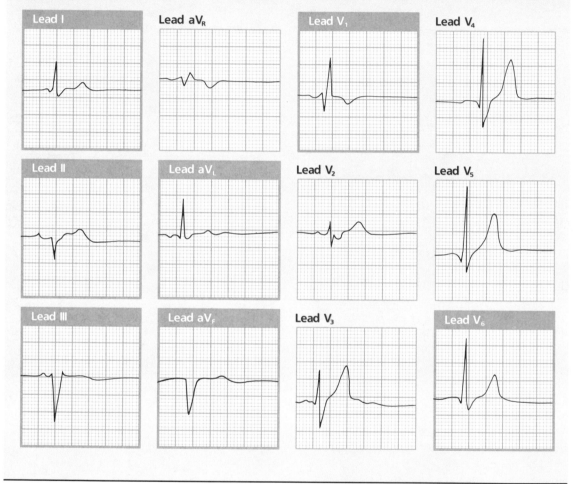

tion of the characteristics that signify the two abnormalities:
• in lead V_1, an rSR' pattern
• in lead V_6, a qRs pattern
• in leads II, III, and aV_F, a qR pattern
• in leads I and aV_L, an rS pattern
• right axis deviation.
(See *Recognizing bifascicular block: RBBB and LPHB*.)

Trifascicular block

In a trifascicular block, all three of the ventricular fascicles are blocked—a condition known as complete heart block. If one of the three fascicles is only partially blocked, the ECG will show a bifascicular block and a first-degree AV block.

For more information on AV blocks, see Chapter 4.

Recognizing bifascicular block: RBBB and LPHB

This 12-lead electrocardiogram shows characteristic changes of a bifascicular block consisting of right bundle-branch block (RBBB) and left posterior hemiblock (LPHB). The rSR' pattern in lead V_1 and the qRs pattern in lead V_6 indicate RBBB. The qR pattern in leads II, III, and aV_F and the rS pattern in leads I and aV_L indicate LPHB.

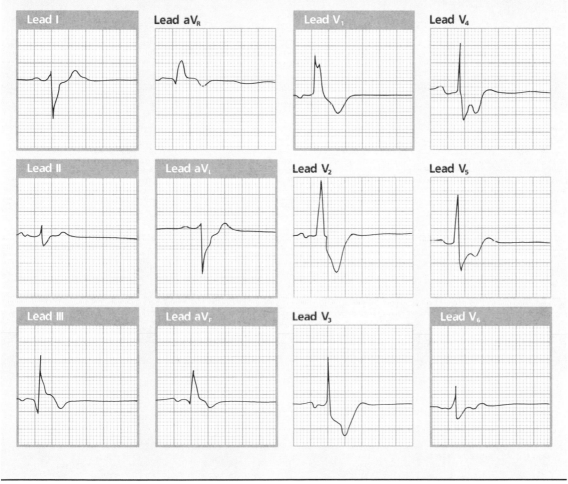

Treatment

With a single fascicular block, treatment is typically aimed at the underlying condition. Usually, you'll also monitor the block in case it becomes more extensive.

When an RBBB occurs after an anterior wall MI, some doctors insert a temporary transvenous pacemaker as a prophylactic measure. Hemiblocks usually don't produce symptoms, unless another interventricular conduction block is present.

When a bifascicular block occurs soon after an acute MI, the doctor may insert a temporary transvenous pacemaker. When a trifascicular block is associated with an acute MI or hemodynamic instability, the doctor will insert a temporary transvenous pacemaker.

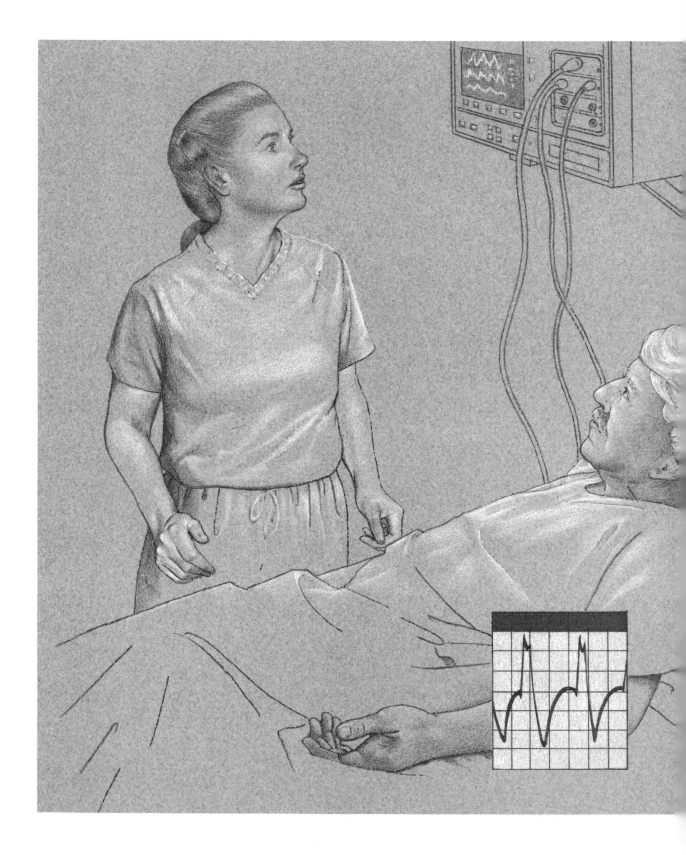

CHAPTER 10

Tachycardias

Tachycardia poses a serious threat because cardiac output may plummet, triggering hemodynamic instability. As the ventricular rate rises above normal, the amount of time that blood can flow into the ventricles — known as ventricular filling time — shortens. Thus, less blood flows into the ventricles between contractions. And, of course, less blood is ejected with each contraction.

This reduction in the amount of blood ejected per contraction, known as stroke volume, doesn't automatically reduce cardiac output. That's because cardiac output — the amount of blood ejected per minute — is determined by both stroke volume and ventricular rate. You'll see this relationship expressed in the formula: cardiac output = stroke volume × ventricular rate.

So even though the heart is pumping less blood per contraction than normal, it's also contracting more times per minute than normal. The result: Cardiac output remains normal.

But this occurs only if the ventricles are healthy—*and* only up to a point. If, for instance, the ventricular rate suddenly rises above 150 beats/minute, even a healthy heart won't be able to compensate. Cardiac output will fall, and hemodynamic instability will develop.

Given these implications of tachycardia, you need to know how to identify it and how to intervene quickly and confidently. As you'll see, how you treat tachycardia depends on the type of tachycardia your patient has. And your ability to identify the various types of narrow and wide QRS-complex tachycardias depends on your electrocardiogram (ECG) interpretation skills.

In this chapter, you'll find the information you need to identify and treat the various types of tachycardias. The chapter consists of two main sections—the first covering five types of narrow QRS-complex tachycardias, the second covering two types of wide QRS-complex tachycardias. For each type, you'll find relevant information on causes, assessment findings, ECG characteristics, and treatment.

Narrow QRS-complex tachycardias

The term *narrow QRS complex* is somewhat misleading. Actually, the QRS complex isn't abnormally narrow; it's normal. Thus, with these tachycardias, the duration of the QRS complex (and of ventricular depolarization) is within normal limits. The QRS complex is "narrow" only when compared with the wide QRS complex that characterizes the tachycardias discussed in the second half of this chapter.

All narrow QRS-complex tachycardias are supraventricular tachycardias (SVTs)—that is, the abnormal impulse originates above the ventricles. The impulse may begin in the sinoatrial node, the atria, or the atrioventricular (AV) node. The impulse then travels through the heart's conduction system depolarizing both ventricles simultaneously—and producing a narrow QRS complex.

Characteristic ECG changes

When you see a QRS complex with a normal duration (0.04 to 0.10 second), you know that the impulse originates above the ventricles. When a patient has narrow QRS-complex tachycardia, however, the complexes will also be close together. Sometimes they're so close that only a single wave is visible between them. This is probably a T wave, but it could be a P wave that's visible because the T wave may be almost flat. Without a baseline between QRS complexes, you can't confidently identify it as either a P wave or a T wave.

Thus, the general characteristics of narrow QRS-complex tachycardia are:
• a ventricular rate greater than 100 beats/minute
• a regular ventricular rhythm
• a normal-width QRS complex
• one wave between QRS complexes with no visible baseline. (See *Identifying narrow QRS-complex tachycardia.*)

Types of narrow QRS-complex tachycardias

Narrow QRS-complex tachycardias are classified by the rhythms that cause them. Thus, the primary types of narrow QRS-complex tachycardias include:
• AV nodal reentry tachycardia
• circus movement tachycardia
• atrial tachycardia with a 1:1 conduction to the ventricles
• atrial flutter with a 2:1 ratio or a varying ratio close to 2:1
• atrial fibrillation with rapid ventricular response
• paroxysmal sinus tachycardia.

Because the last type is rare, it won't be covered in the discussion below.

AV nodal reentry tachycardia
This narrow QRS-complex tachycardia is by far the most common. In fact, it accounts for about half of all narrow QRS-complex tachycardias.

Identifying narrow QRS-complex tachycardia

This rhythm strip shows the characteristics of narrow QRS-complex tachycardia. Note the ventricular rate of 240, the regular ventricular rhythm, the normal-width QRS complexes, and the single wave between QRS complexes.

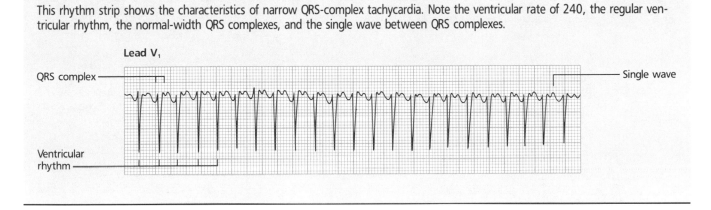

Lead V₁

QRS complex

Single wave

Ventricular rhythm

Produced by a short circuit in the AV node, this type of tachycardia is characterized by ventricular rates between 100 and 280 beats/minute, with about 170 beats/minute the average. Usually transient, AV nodal reentry tachycardia may also be sustained and resistant to traditional medical interventions.

Causes

Typically, this type of tachycardia occurs in patients with healthy hearts, not in those with organic heart disease. How, though, does the reentry occur? To begin, the AV node consists of a network of conductive tissue. Some of these interconnecting pathways have slow conduction with fast recovery (a short refractory period). Other pathways have fast conduction with slow recovery (a long refractory period). The difference between these pathways provides the right environment for a reentry circuit. Normally, the impulse reaches the AV node and travels via the fast pathway, resulting in a normal PR interval on the ECG.

An episode of AV nodal reentry tachycardia begins when a premature atrial contraction (PAC) finds the fast pathway refractory. The impulse then travels down the slow pathway to the bundle of His. As the impulse enters the bundle of His, it also travels in a retrograde direction up the fast pathway within the repolarized AV node, reentering the atrial tissue.

When the slow AV node pathway is ready to conduct again, the impulse comes around, and the reentry continues. The atria and ventricles are then repeatedly stimulated simultaneously. (See *Understanding AV nodal reentry,* page 136.)

Assessment findings

Because the atria and ventricles contract simultaneously (or almost simultaneously), the right atrium can't pump blood through the closed tricuspid valve. Instead, the blood is forced back into the superior vena cava, producing a regular, rapid, visible pulsation of the external jugular veins. Because this visible pulsing in the neck resembles the rhythmic puffing of a frog, it's known as the frog sign. This sign signals a diagnosis of AV nodal reentry tachycardia.

With AV nodal reentry tachycardia, the patient's pulse will be normal; his systolic blood pressure, constant; and the loudness of S₁, constant. Because the tachycardia is typically transient, its signs and symptoms—which include hypotension; syncope; cool, clammy skin; and other findings related to decreased cardiac output—usually last only a few seconds to several minutes.

Characteristic ECG changes

The PAC that triggers AV nodal reentry tachycardia has an abnormally long PR interval. Be-

PATHOPHYSIOLOGY

Understanding AV nodal reentry

Use the following illustrations to compare normal conduction through the atrioventricular (AV) node with AV nodal reentry.

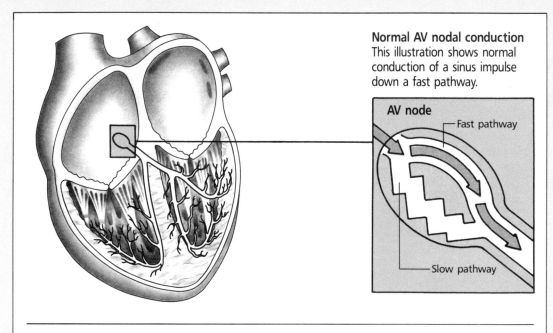

Normal AV nodal conduction
This illustration shows normal conduction of a sinus impulse down a fast pathway.

AV node
Fast pathway
Slow pathway

Progression of AV nodal reentry

In this illustration, a premature atrial contraction with a long PR interval finds the fast pathway refractory and is conducted down a slow pathway of the AV node.

After the impulse traverses the slow pathway, it travels simultaneously into the ventricles and up the fast pathway to the atria.

The impulse's return to the atria via the fast pathway and to the ventricles via the slow pathway establishes a reentry circuit, which causes repeated, simultaneous stimulation of the atria and ventricles.

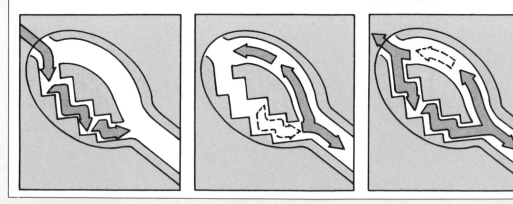

Recognizing AV nodal reentry tachycardia

This 12-lead electrocardiogram shows characteristic findings of an atrioventricular (AV) nodal reentry tachycardia. Note that the P waves peek out of the ends of the QRS complexes in leads II, III, and aV_F.

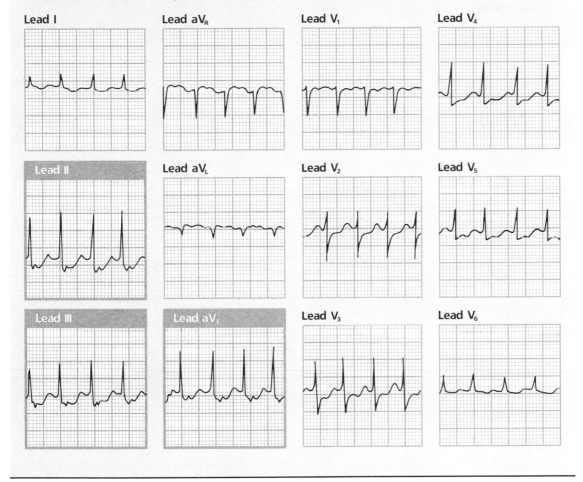

Lead I   Lead aV_R Lead V_1 Lead V_4

Lead II   Lead aV_L Lead V_2 Lead V_5

Lead III   Lead aV_F Lead V_3 Lead V_6

cause the impulse travels in a loop within the AV node, producing simultaneous depolarization of the atria and ventricles, the P wave is usually hidden in the QRS complex during the tachycardia. Many times, you may see the P wave peeking out of the terminal portion of the QRS complex. Always compare the terminal portion of the QRS complex during the underlying rhythm with that during the tachycardia. This P wave distorts the QRS complex and can be mistaken for an r wave in lead MCL_1 (V_1) or for an s wave in leads II, III, and aV_F. (See *Recognizing AV nodal reentry tachycardia*.)

Treatment

AV nodal reentry tachycardia can be terminated with a vagal maneuver, cardioversion, or I.V. administration of adenosine or verapamil. These interventions alter the refractory state of the pathways in the AV node, interrupting the reentry circuit.

When AV nodal reentry tachycardia proves resistant to medical therapy, either surgery or

PATHOPHYSIOLOGY

Understanding CMT

Use these two illustrations to review how circus movement tachycardia (CMT) occurs in patients with an accessory pathway joining the atria and the ventricles.

A premature atrial contraction finds the accessory pathway refractory and then travels down to the ventricles via the atrioventricular (AV) node.

The impulse simultaneously stimulates the ventricles via the normal conduction system and stimulates the atria via the accessory pathway.

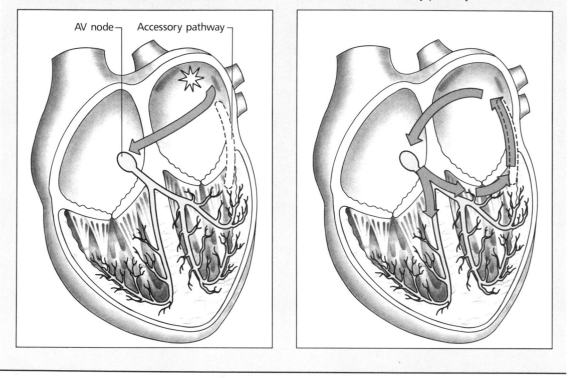

a radio frequency current may be used to ablate the AV node, which is then replaced with a permanent pacemaker. As an alternative, surgery or a radio frequency current can be used to ablate just one of the AV pathways, thus halting the reentry circuit but retaining normal conduction to the ventricles.

Circus movement tachycardia

Circus movement tachycardia (CMT) accounts for about 40% of all narrow QRS-complex tachycardias. Like AV nodal reentry tachycardia, it results from an electrical impulse being caught in a short circuit. CMT may produce between 150 and 250 beats/minute, with about 170 beats/minute the average. CMT is the most common arrhythmia detected in patients with Wolff-Parkinson-White syndrome.

Causes

This abnormality occurs in patients, such as those with Wolff-Parkinson-White syndrome, who have an accessory pathway (an abnormal band of conductive tissue) joining the atria and the ventricles. (See *Understanding CMT* and *Understanding a delta wave.*)

The circus movement begins when a PAC reaches the accessory pathway when it's refractory. The impulse traverses the AV node and the rest of the conduction system as usual. When the impulse depolarizes the ventricles, it also moves to the ventricular end of the accessory pathway, which can now conduct it. Thus, the impulse moves in a retrograde manner into the atria, which depolarize again as the impulse reaches the AV node and repeats its trip through the conduction system. As the ventricles begin to depolarize once more, the impulse again travels up the accessory pathway, reentering the atria. The cycle continues regularly and rapidly.

Significance
Although CMT itself is fairly easy to treat, the preexisting condition that permits this tachycardia — the accessory pathway — presents the real danger. That's because patients with CMT seem to be prone to atrial fibrillation. And the accessory pathway doesn't protect the ventricles as a healthy AV node does.

A healthy AV node can control the ventricular rate, despite a bombardment of impulses from the atria. But an accessory pathway simply conducts the impulses from the atria — no matter how many. When atrial fibrillation occurs in a patient with an accessory pathway, he's at risk for ventricular fibrillation.

Assessment findings
Like AV nodal reentry tachycardia, CMT produces the frog sign. Similarly, the patient will have a regular pulse, a constant systolic blood pressure, and a constant S_1.

Characteristic ECG changes
Like AV nodal reentry tachycardia, CMT occurs paroxysmally. But in CMT the initiating PAC produces a normal PR interval. That's because after the PAC finds the accessory pathway refractory, it travels through the normal conduction system without delay.

The ventricles are depolarized simultaneously and, of course, the QRS complex has a normal duration. Atrial and ventricular depolarization occur sequentially in CMT, so the P waves and QRS complexes appear separately

Understanding a delta wave

In patients with Wolff-Parkinson-White syndrome, the sinus impulse reaches the ventricle via an accessory pathway outside the normal conduction system. This abnormally conducted impulse causes the ventricular myocardium to depolarize earlier than normal. A delta wave, or slur, appears on the electrocardiogram at the beginning of the QRS complex.

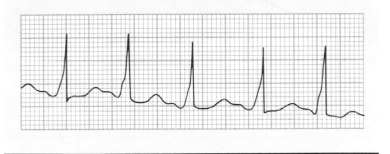

on the ECG. However, the P waves will appear closer to the preceding QRS complexes than to the succeeding ones. P waves usually are inverted in leads II, III, and aV_r.

In about 30% of patients, QRS complex alternans occurs. With this abnormality, every other QRS complex is shorter than the preceding one. Because alternans occurs at the beginning of all SVTs, it's a valid diagnostic clue only when it continues beyond the first 5 seconds of the tachycardia. (See *Recognizing CMT,* page 140.)

Treatment
A vagal maneuver, cardioversion, or I.V. administration of certain drugs — in particular, adenosine and procainamide — may be used to terminate a CMT. The drugs used most often to treat tachycardia — verapamil and digoxin — are contraindicated for CMT. That's because they shorten the refractory period of the accessory pathway, allowing even more impulses to reach the ventricles. This can lead to ventricular rates over 300 beats/minute and, ultimately, to ventricular fibrillation.

Recognizing CMT

This 12-lead electrocardiogram shows circus movement tachycardia (CMT). Note the normal PR interval, the narrow (or normal) QRS complex, the heart rate of approximately 160 beats/minute, and the regular rhythm. The inverted P wave in the ST segment in leads II, III, and aV$_F$ differentiates this tachycardia from an atrioventricular nodal reentry tachycardia.

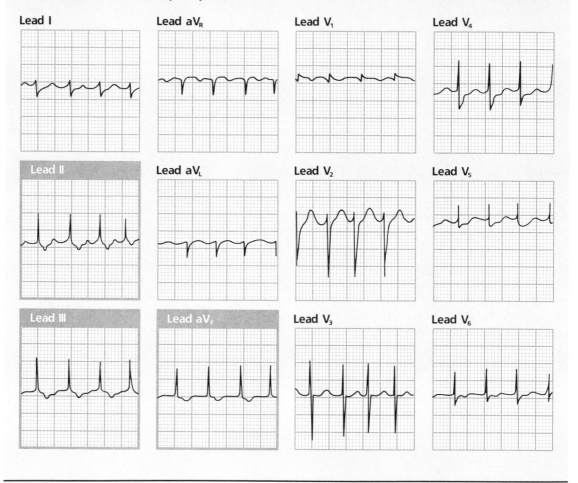

Atrial tachycardia

Atrial tachycardia triggers SVT only when the AV node fails to block some of the atrial impulses. Usually, atrial tachycardia is associated with an atrial rate-ventricular rate ratio of 2:1 or higher. Thus, despite atrial tachycardia, the ventricular rate remains within the normal range. If, however, the AV node conducts every impulse (150 to 250 beats/minute) to the ven-

tricles, the resulting rapid ventricular rate may cause hemodynamic compromise.

Causes

Paroxysmal atrial tachycardia usually stems from reentry within ischemic atrial tissue. Typically, the ischemia results from coronary artery disease (CAD).

Recognizing atrial tachycardia

This 12-lead electrocardiogram shows a narrow QRS-complex tachycardia resulting from atrial tachycardia. Note that the atrial and ventricular rates are 150 beats/minute. P waves are inverted in leads I and aV_L and are upright in aV_R. This suggests that the impulse originated in the inferior area of the left atrium.

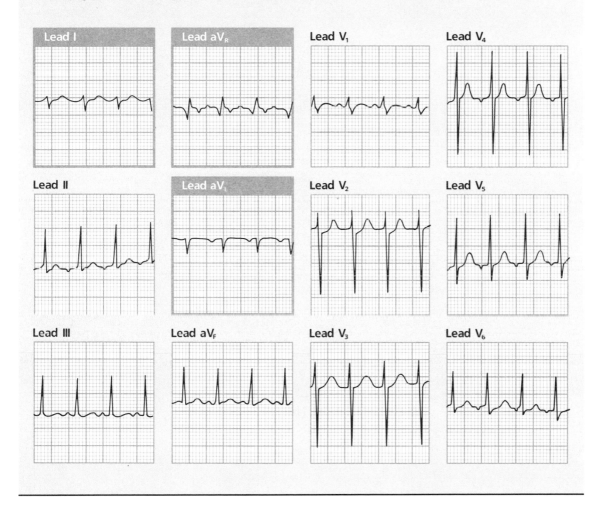

Nonparoxysmal atrial tachycardia may result when digitalis toxicity triggers delayed after-depolarization.

Assessment findings
When atrial tachycardia causes narrow QRS-complex tachycardia, the patient will have a regular pulse and a constant (though not necessarily acceptable) systolic blood pressure.

Also, you won't see neck vein pulsations, and S_1 will remain constant.

Characteristic ECG changes
Atrial tachycardia is usually initiated by a PAC; the atrial rate then continues at 140 to 250 beats/minute. The ventricular rate depends upon the condition of the AV node.

The distinguishing feature of atrial tachycardia is its P-wave morphology. Impulses arising

Recognizing atrial flutter

This 12-lead electrocardiogram shows atrial flutter with a 2:1 conduction ratio in leads I, II, III, and V$_1$ through V$_6$. Also, note that as the conduction ratio changes in lead aV$_F$, the flutter waves become more visible.

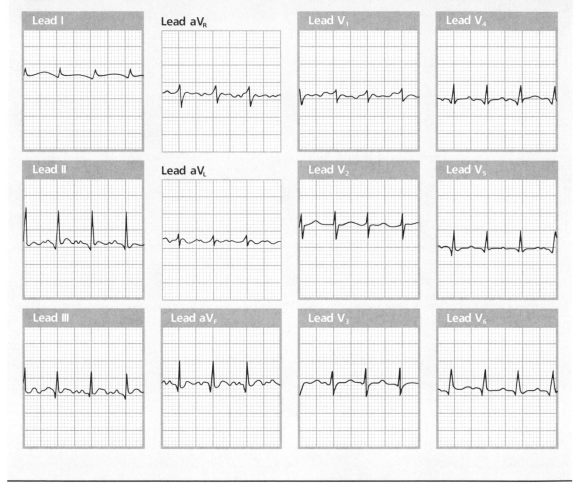

from the right atrium show inverted P waves in leads aV$_R$ and upright P waves in leads I and aV$_L$. Impulses arising from the left atrium show inverted P waves in leads I and aV$_L$ and upright P waves in aV$_R$. (See *Recognizing atrial tachycardia*, page 141.)

Treatment
Because the AV node isn't involved in this narrow QRS-complex tachycardia, the drugs and vagal maneuvers that can convert AV nodal

reentry tachycardia and CMT are seldom effective. At best, these interventions temporarily slow the ventricular rate by blocking the AV node. If the rhythm doesn't convert spontaneously, especially in a symptomatic patient, cardioversion is necessary.

When atrial tachycardia results from digitalis toxicity, treat the underlying problem first.

Recognizing atrial fibrillation

This 12-lead electrocardiogram shows narrow QRS-complex tachycardia from atrial fibrillation. Note that in all leads no identifiable P waves appear. Also, the ventricular rhythm is rapid and irregular.

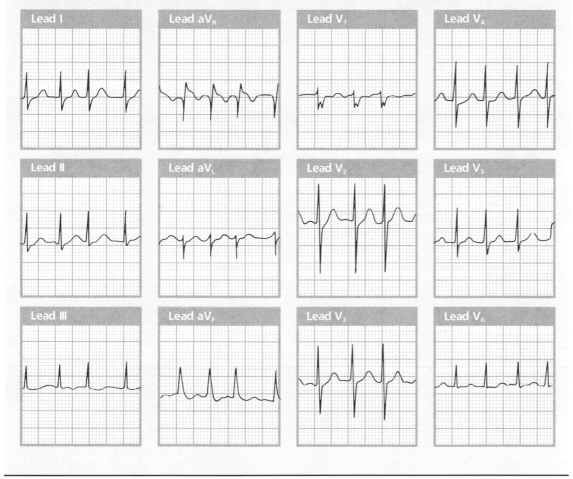

Atrial flutter

Atrial flutter is characterized by an atrial rate between 250 and 400 beats/minute. As with atrial tachycardia, if the AV node can't block enough atrial impulses to maintain a normal ventricular rate, a narrow QRS-complex tachycardia results. As with any such tachycardia, the decreased ventricular filling may reduce cardiac output.

Causes

Atrial flutter is thought to result from reentry within atrial tissue affected by CAD. When the AV node is influenced by catecholamines or other stimulating forces, the rapid atrial rate is conducted more readily to the ventricles.

Assessment findings

If the ratio of atrial beats to ventricular beats is 2:1, the patient's pulse will be regular, and his systolic blood pressure will be constant. If the ratio varies, his pulse and systolic blood

Monitoring narrow QRS-complex tachycardia

To monitor a patient with narrow QRS-complex tachycardia, select the lead that best shows the P wave. Usually, this will be lead II, though V₁ (MCL₁) may also give you a good view of the P wave.

AV nodal reentry tachycardia
In atrioventricular nodal reentry tachycardia, the P wave may peek out at the end of the QRS complex in lead II, as shown here. To detect this P wave, compare the terminal portion of the QRS complex during the underlying rhythm with the terminal portion of the QRS complex during the tachycardia.

Lead II

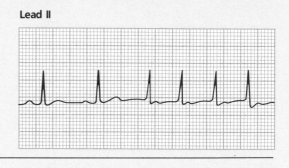

Circus movement tachycardia
In circus movement tachycardia, the P waves and QRS complexes are separate; however, the P wave is closer to the preceding QRS complex than the following one. This waveform also shows QRS complex alternans.

Lead II

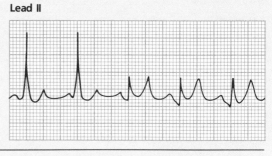

Atrial flutter
In atrial flutter, you'll see sawtooth P waves in lead II.

Lead II

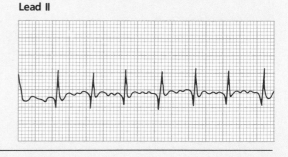

Atrial fibrillation
In atrial fibrillation, the P waves can't be identified, and the R-R interval is irregular.

Lead II

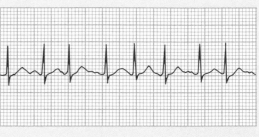

pressure will be irregular. When you observe the patient's neck veins, you'll see flutter waves; that is, slight, rapid, regular pulsations. S₁ will be constant.

Characteristic ECG changes
Flutter waves—called sawtooth waves because of their appearance in some leads—occur regularly at a rate of 250 to 400/minute and are visible when the conduction ratio is greater than 2:1. When the ratio is 2:1, identifying atrial flutter as the cause of ventricular tachycardia is more difficult. But if you note pointed P waves, look at the end of the QRS complex and at the T wave for the same pointed shape. If you note that the peaks of the clearly identified P waves and the partially hidden ones plot out regularly across the strip, at a rate of 250 to 400 beats/minute, suspect atrial flutter. (See *Recognizing atrial flutter*, page 142.)

Treatment
As with atrial tachycardia, atrial flutter usually can't be corrected by using drugs or vagal maneuvers. Typically, cardioversion is necessary to convert this arrhythmia to a normal sinus rhythm if the arrhythmia doesn't convert spontaneously.

Atrial fibrillation
In atrial fibrillation, the atrial rate ranges from 400 to 600 beats/minute, causing the atria to quiver instead of contracting regularly. When the AV node can't protect the ventricles adequately—for example, due to ischemia—a rapid ventricular rate develops.

Atrial fibrillation itself eliminates atrial kick, thus reducing the amount of blood delivered to the ventricles. Add to this a rapid ventricular rate, and you can see why cardiac output drops significantly. Atrial fibrillation also poses the risk of mural thrombi from stagnant blood lining the walls of the quivering, non-contractile atria.

Causes
Atrial fibrillation results from many circus reentry pathways in the atria. Chronic obstructive pulmonary disease, congestive heart failure, CAD, and stimulants, such as caffeine and nico-

tine, can cause atrial irritability. Ischemia or metabolic influences can transform atrial cells from nonpacemaker to pacemaker by altering the cell membrane in one of two ways: The resting membrane can be made less negative or the fast sodium channels may be deactivated, leaving only the slow sodium/calcium channels in operation and giving the atrial cells the property of automaticity.

Assessment findings
In a patient with narrow QRS-complex tachycardia resulting from atrial fibrillation, you'll note an irregular pulse and irregular neck vein pulsations. The patient's systolic blood pressure and the loudness of S₁ will vary.

Characteristic ECG changes
Atrial fibrillation produces no identifiable P waves. The irregularity of the ventricular rhythm distinguishes this condition from other narrow QRS-complex tachycardias, but the rapidity of the rhythm may make identification difficult. If vagal maneuvers or certain drugs are used to block AV node conduction, the temporary slowing of the ventricular rate may make identification easier. (See *Recognizing atrial fibrillation*, page 143.)

Treatment
Usually, cardioversion is required to terminate this rhythm.

Monitoring patients

To monitor a patient who has a narrow QRS-complex tachycardia, you may select either lead II or lead V₁ (MCL₁). (See *Monitoring narrow QRS-complex tachycardia*.)

Wide QRS-complex tachycardias

With these tachycardias, the ventricles take longer than normal to depolarize (over 0.10 second), making the QRS complex abnormally

PATHOPHYSIOLOGY

How ventricular rhythms cause wide QRS-complex tachycardia

With this arrhythmia, an ectopic impulse originates in one ventricle and depolarizes it, as shown.

Then the electrical impulse travels to the other ventricle, depolarizing it. The result of this sequential depolarization is a wide QRS complex.

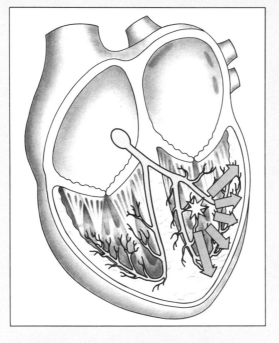

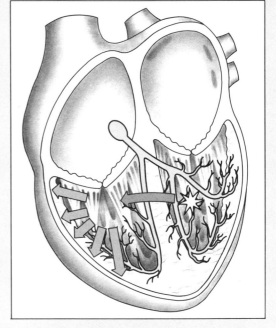

wide. Unlike narrow QRS-complex tachycardias, which all originate above the ventricles, wide QRS-complex tachycardias may originate above the ventricles or in them. And because giving the appropriate treatment depends on knowing the origin of the impulse, you must be able to distinguish these two groups of wide QRS-complex tachycardias.

The leads that provide the most useful information for identifying the wide QRS-complex tachycardias are V_1 and V_6. These leads demonstrate the morphologic features that research has identified to differentiate between ventricular tachycardias and SVT. You can also use the bipolar versions of these leads, MCL_1 and MCL_6.

Types of wide QRS-complex tachycardias

Wide QRS-complex tachycardias are usually classified more broadly than narrow QRS-complex tachycardias. Whereas the narrow QRS-complex tachycardias are classified by the specific underlying arrhythmia or the abnormal mechanism, the wide QRS-complex tachycardias are classified only as either ventricular rhythms (those originating in the ventricles) or supraventricular rhythms (those originating above the ventricles).

To distinguish these two types, you'll use your assessment findings as well as your interpretation of the patient's ECG. For instance, you'll examine the width, shape, and deflection

Understanding torsades de pointes

In this ventricular tachycardia, the QRS complex changes its shape and is sometimes negative, sometimes positive. Characterized by a ventricular rate ranging from 150 to 250 beats/minute, torsades de pointes (twisting of the points) may stop and start suddenly. Sometimes the sinus rhythm resumes spontaneously, but in other cases, torsades de pointes degenerates into ventricular fibrillation. Frequently, the onset follows a long-short cycle sequence.

Any condition that may cause a prolonged QT interval can trigger torsades de pointes. These conditions include congenital prolonged QT syndrome (Romano-Ward syndrome), myocardial ischemia, sinoatrial disease that results in profound bradycardia, the vagal response, subarachnoid hemorrhage, atrioventricular block, and Prinzmetal's angina. The arrhythmia may also result from electrolyte imbalances (hypokalemia, hypocalcemia, or hypomagnesemia), drug toxicity (particularly from quinidine, procainamide, disopyramide, or amiodarone), and overdoses of certain psychotropic drugs (such as phenothiazines and tricyclic antidepressants).

ECG interpretation
On the strip below, note the following characteristics:
• changing direction of QRS complex
• long-short cycle
• prolonged QT interval.

Treatment
If the patient with torsades has no pulse, use cardiopulmonary resuscitation. If he's unstable, use cardioversion.

If the patient is stable, follow these steps. Continue following them only as long as the arrhythmia persists.
• Administer 1 to 2 g of magnesium chloride or magnesium sulfate by I.V. bolus over 5 minutes. Then begin a continuous drip of 1 to 2 g/hour for 4 to 6 hours. You should give magnesium even if the patient has a normal serum magnesium level.
• Use atrial pacing at 90 to 110 beats/minute. Or administer 100 mg of isoproterenol I.V. over 5 minutes, up to a maximum of 1 g. These interventions should increase the patient's heart rate and shorten the QT interval.
• If the patient is hypokalemic, give potassium chloride.

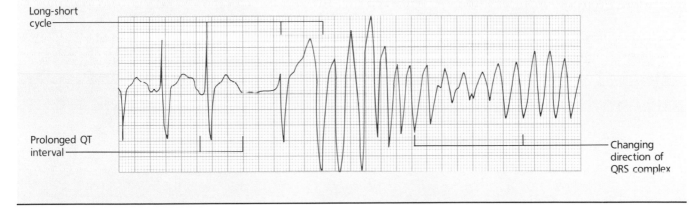

of the QRS complex and other characteristics such as the ventricular rhythm and rate.

Ventricular tachycardia
In this type of tachycardia, an impulse originates in one of the ventricles and depolarizes it first. The impulse is then conducted to the other ventricle and depolarizes it. This delayed, sequential (rather than simultaneous) depolarization of the ventricles produces the wide QRS complex. (See *How ventricular rhythms cause wide QRS-complex tachycardia.*)

Assessment findings
About 50% of patients with this type of tachycardia will show signs of AV dissociation. These signs include random, intermittent neck vein pulsations; a varying intensity of the radial pulse; and a varying intensity of S_1.

The random, intermittent neck vein pulsations result when the atria and ventricles,

Wide QRS-complex tachycardia: Ventricular origin

Both these 12-lead electrocardiograms (ECGs) show wide QRS-complex tachycardia originating in the ventricles. On the ECG on this page, the deflection of the QRS complex in lead V_1 is positive and biphasic. Other key ECG characteristics include a QRS complex with a negative deflection and an extreme electrical axis deviation in lead V_6.

Positive QRS-complex deflection in lead V_1

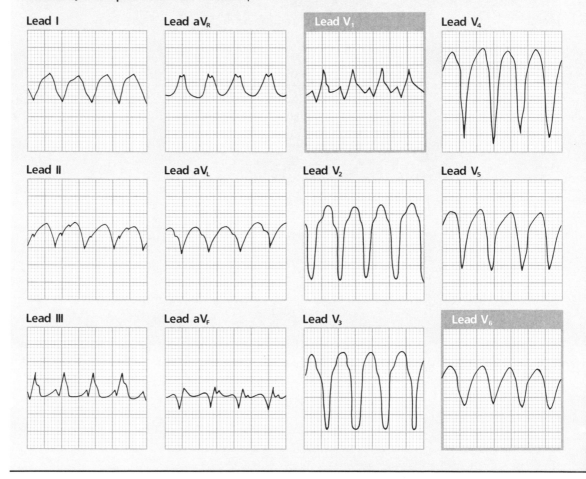

which are contracting independently, happen to contract simultaneously. The blood from the right atrium—unable to traverse a closed tricuspid valve—is forced to travel back up into the superior vena cava, causing the random pulsation.

The independent beating of the atria and ventricles also produces a varying intensity of the radial pulse. With each atrial contraction, the ventricles receive a different volume of blood. Thus, end-diastolic volume—and the volume of blood actually leaving the ventricles—varies with each ventricular systole. Also, the varying end-diastolic volume produces differing degrees of stretch in the ventricular wall. And the more the myocardial fibers stretch, the greater the force of contraction. So, the

Unlike the first 12-lead ECG, this one shows a QRS complex in lead V_1 with a negative deflection. Other characteristics that identify the arrhythmia as having a ventricular origin include a broad R wave in leads V_1 and V_2, a slurred S wave in lead V_1, and a delay from the beginning of the QRS complex to the low point of the S wave in leads V_1 and V_2.

Negative QRS-complex deflection in lead V_1

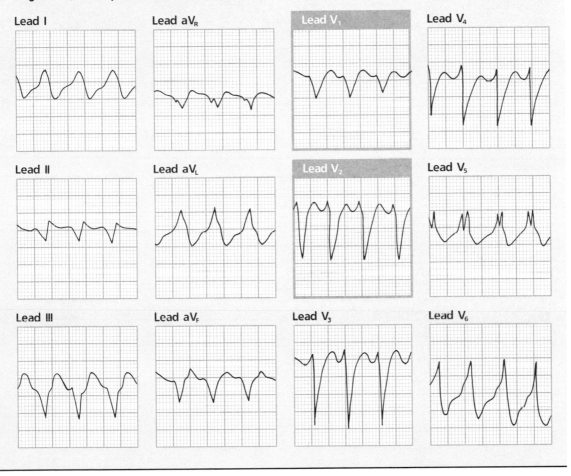

greater the end-diastolic volume, the stronger the patient's radial pulse.

Varying heart sounds also result from varying end-diastolic volume. That's because this changing volume varies the forcefulness of the mitral and tricuspid valve closures. And, of course, these closures at the beginning of ventricular systole produce S_1.

Characteristic ECG changes

By definition, all wide QRS-complex tachycardias have complexes wider than the normal 0.04 to 0.10 second. When the tachycardia originates in the ventricular tissue, the QRS complex can measure 0.14 second or more—especially if it has a positive deflection in lead V_1. In torsades de pointes, a variation of ventricular tachycardia, the QRS complex may fluc-

PATHOPHYSIOLOGY

How supraventricular rhythms cause wide QRS-complex tachycardia

The illustrations below show one way in which a supraventricular rhythm can cause wide QRS-complex tachycardia.

In the first illustration, a supraventricular impulse travels down the left bundle branch but finds the right bundle branch blocked.

After the impulse depolarizes the left ventricle, it travels to the right ventricle and depolarizes it. This sequential ventricular depolarization produces a wide QRS complex.

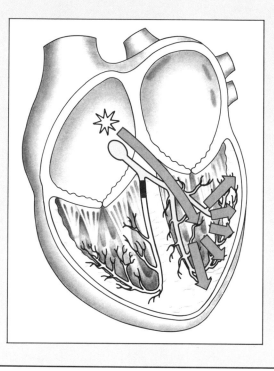

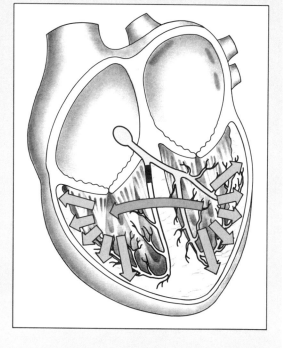

tuate between being positive and negative. (See *Understanding torsades de pointes*, page 147.)

Deflection. Once you've established that the QRS complex is wide, note its deflection and shape (or morphology).

If the QRS complex is mainly positive in lead V_1, is it monophasic, biphasic, or triphasic? If it's monophasic or biphasic, the rhythm is most likely ventricular, not supraventricular.

With a biphasic r wave, note whether it has a notched top producing two peaks. If the

left peak is taller than the right peak, the rhythm originates in the ventricles. If the right peak is taller than the left peak, the rhythm may be ventricular or supraventricular. If V_6 is mainly negative, the rhythm is ventricular.

If the QRS complex is mainly negative in lead V_1, look for the following additional characteristics:
• an initial r wave in either V_1 or V_2 greater than 0.03 second
• a slurring or notching of the downstroke of the S wave in either V_1 or V_2
• a duration of 0.06 second or greater from

Wide QRS-complex tachycardia: Supraventricular origin

This 12-lead electrocardiogram shows wide QRS-complex tachycardia originating above the ventricles. In lead V_1, the deflection of the QRS complex is negative. But also in this lead, the r wave is less than 0.03 second, the duration from the r wave to the peak of the S wave is less than 0.06 second, and the S wave has a clean downstroke. These findings rule out ventricular tachycardia. Also, note the absence of P waves and the irregular ventricular rhythm.

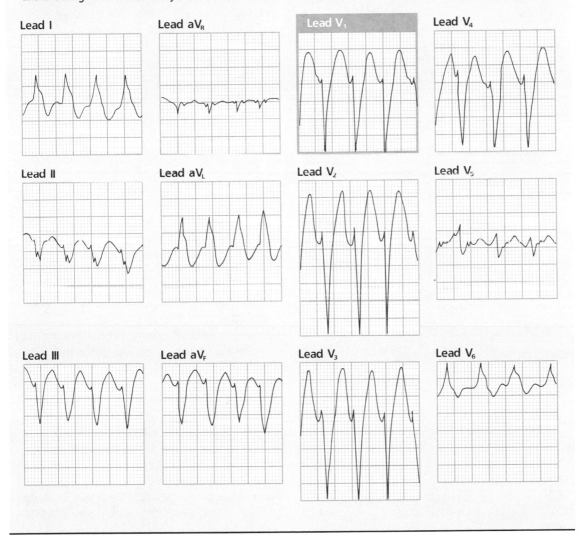

the beginning of the QRS complex to the peak of the S wave in any lead
• any Q wave in lead V_6.

Any of these four findings strongly suggests a ventricular origin. However, if none of these findings are present, then suspect SVT.

Concordance. The term concordance refers to a pattern of all positive or all negative QRS complexes in the six precordial leads. Positive concordance often, but not always, indicates a ventricular origin. Negative concordance always indicates a ventricular origin.

Monitoring wide QRS-complex tachycardia

When monitoring a patient with a history of wide QRS-complex tachycardia, use lead V₁ to differentiate ventricular tachycardia from supraventricular tachycardia.

Positive QRS complex
When the QRS complex is positive in lead V₁, the rhythm is probably ventricular if it's monophasic or biphasic with the left peak taller than the right.

Lead V₁

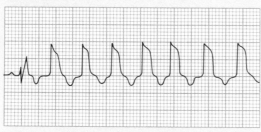

Negative QRS complex
When the QRS complex is negative in lead V₁, the rhythm is probably ventricular if it has an R wave greater than 0.03 second, a slurred S wave, and a delayed low point greater than 0.06 second.

Lead V₁

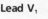

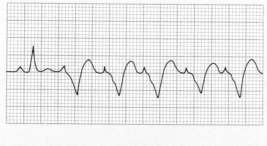

Electrical axis. When the deflection of the QRS complex in leads I, II, and V₆ is negative, an extreme axis deviation (−90 to 180 degrees) indicates a ventricular rhythm.

Rhythm. Usually, the rhythm will be regular. You may note a slight irregularity because ventricular foci aren't dependable.

AV dissociation. With patients who have AV dissociation, you'll note P waves appearing randomly around the QRS complex. If you can find two consecutive P waves, measure the distance between them, and check the atrial rate and rhythm. The rate should be normal and the rhythm should be regular.

Capture beats and fusion beats. With AV dissociation, an occasional sinus impulse may make it to the ventricles and initiate depolarization. If this impulse completely depolarizes the ventricles before the ventricles initiate the next ectopic impulse, a capture beat results. If the sinus impulse and the ectopic impulse depolarize the ventricles simultaneously, a fusion beat results.

Capture beats and fusion beats have QRS complexes that are smaller and narrower than those of the rest of the tachycardia. These beats don't occur very often. (See *Wide QRS-complex tachycardia: Ventricular origin*, pages 148 and 149.)

Supraventricular rhythms
Most supraventricular rhythms reach the ventricles simultaneously by way of the bundle branches and thus produce a narrow QRS-complex tachycardia. But when the patient has a pathologic bundle-branch block, the supraventricular impulse will reach one ventricle first, then the other. Such sequential depolarization also occurs when the supraventricular impulse finds one of the bundle branches refractory. In either case, the delayed ventricular depolarization produces a wide QRS complex. (See *How supraventricular rhythms cause wide QRS-complex tachycardia*, page 150.)

Assessment findings
Your assessment findings will depend on the exact source of the supraventricular rhythm. Your findings will differ, for instance, depending on whether sinus tachycardia, atrial tachycardia, or AV nodal reentry tachycardia is

producing the rapid ventricular rate. Your findings will also depend on whether or not your patient has a bundle-branch block.

Characteristic ECG changes
Typically, the QRS complex will measure between 0.10 and 0.12 second.

Deflection. Again, once you've established that the QRS complex is wide, note its deflection and morphology. If the QRS complex is mainly positive in lead V_1, note whether it's monophasic, biphasic, or triphasic. If it's triphasic, the rhythm is most likely supraventricular.

If you note a positive QRS complex in lead V_6, the arrhythmia probably originates above the ventricles.

Rhythm. Usually a supraventricular rhythm will be regular. An irregular rhythm generally indicates atrial fibrillation with a bundle-branch block or conduction over an accessory pathway, or atrial flutter with a bundle-branch block and varying AV conduction.

P wave. You won't see P waves on the ECG, even though atrial activity is occurring. (See *Wide QRS-complex tachycardia: Supraventricular origin,* page 151.)

Treatment

When a patient suddenly develops wide QRS-complex tachycardia, you need to respond at once. If possible, record a 12-lead ECG. If you can't run a 12-lead ECG, record leads I, II, MCL_1, and MCL_6.

If the patient is hemodynamically unstable, use cardioversion before examining the ECG. Once his rhythm has been converted, you can read the ECG to identify the source of the arrhythmia.

If the patient is hemodynamically stable during the tachycardia, or if his rhythm has been cardioverted but becomes tachycardic again, treat him based on whether the source is ventricular or supraventricular.

Ventricular rhythm
When the patient's wide QRS-complex tachycardia originates in the ventricular tissue, follow the steps below. You should continue following them only as long as the ventricular tachycardia persists.
• Administer 100 mg of procainamide over 5 minutes. (If the patient has an acute myocardial infarction, give lidocaine first.)
• Cardiovert the patient.
• Compare the ECGs showing the tachycardia and the postconversion rhythm.

Supraventricular rhythm
When the patient's wide QRS-complex tachycardia originates above the ventricles, follow one or more of the steps below as ordered. Follow them only as long as the supraventricular tachycardia persists.
• Perform a vagal maneuver.
• Administer 6 mg of adenosine by I.V. push. As necessary, you can give this dose two times.
• Administer 10 mg of verapamil I.V. over 2 to 3 minutes.
• Administer 100 mg of procainamide over 5 minutes.
• Administer a sedative, then use cardioversion.
• Compare the ECGs showing the tachycardia and the postconversion rhythm.

Unknown source
When you're unable to determine whether the wide QRS-complex tachycardia originates in the ventricles or above the ventricles, administer procainamide—not verapamil. However, you shouldn't give procainamide if you suspect torsades de pointes.

Monitoring patients

To monitor a patient who has wide QRS-complex tachycardia, you should select lead V_1 (or MCL_1). (See *Monitoring wide QRS-complex tachycardia.*)

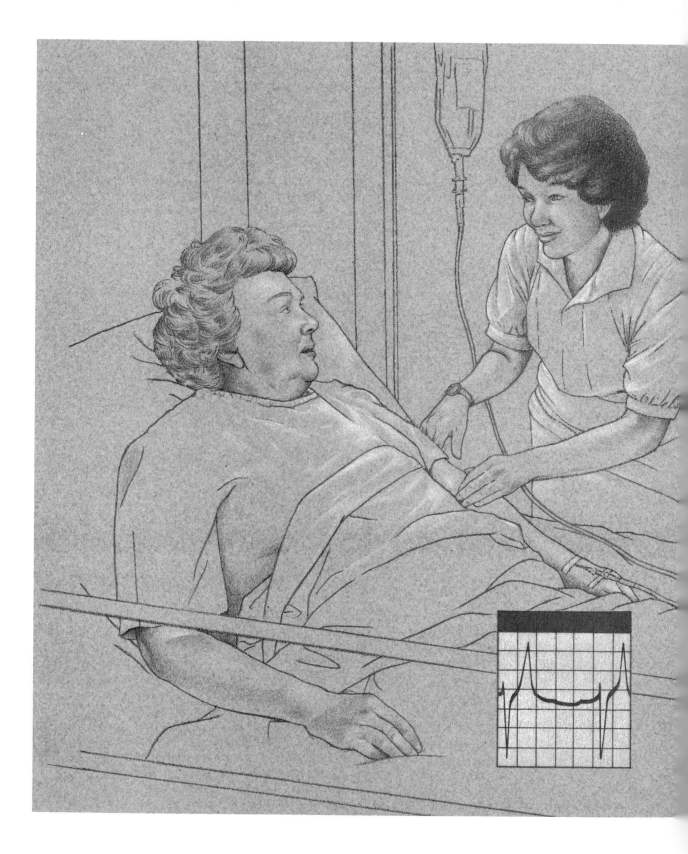

11

Electrolyte disturbances

To function normally, the heart depends on normal electrolyte concentrations. Depolarization results from the cyclic exchange of sodium, potassium, and calcium ions across the cell membrane. And repolarization depends on the sodium-potassium pump, which is regulated by magnesium ions.

Disturbances in electrolyte balance thus affect the myocardial action potential, altering myocardial function and producing changes in the electrocardiogram (ECG). By recognizing these changes early, you can initiate prompt and lifesaving treatment measures.

This chapter will help you identify the ECG changes that typically result from potassium, calcium, and magnesium imbalances. It discusses the common causes of electrolyte disturbances and their effects on myocardial cells. The chapter also points out typical signs and symptoms of electrolyte disturbances and details characteristic ECG changes that appear during cardiac monitoring. Appropriate treatment measures are discussed as well.

Potassium imbalances

In an average-sized person weighing about 155 lb (70 kg), potassium stores total about 3,500 mEq. Normally, intracellular fluid contains about 98% of the body's potassium; extracellular fluid contains only about 2% (3.5 to 5 mEq/liter). The sodium-potassium pump maintains this high intracellular to extracellular ratio. Even small changes in the serum potassium level significantly affect the resting membrane potential, which alters myocardial function.

The kidneys, the primary regulators of potassium homeostasis, control potassium secretion and reabsorption through the renin-angiotensin-aldosterone mechanism. The kidneys also govern renal pH and sodium delivery to the nephrons. When potassium stores overload the system, extrarenal forces trigger the release of insulin and catecholamines, which stimulate potassium uptake by skeletal and cardiac muscles.

Changes in body pH also influence serum potassium levels. Metabolic acidosis creates hyperkalemia because excess hydrogen ions enter the cells, forcing potassium to exit. Conversely, metabolic alkalosis causes hypokalemia because ion shifts are reversed.

Hyperkalemia

In hyperkalemia, the extracellular potassium level rises above 5 mEq/liter, and the intracellular potassium concentration dips. The imbalance may reflect renal failure, metabolic acidosis, trauma, burns, or any illness that compromises renal perfusion or nephron integrity. It also may stem from the use of such agents as potassium supplements, mannitol, angiotensin-converting enzyme inhibitors, cyclosporine, and spironolactone.

Hyperkalemia occurs more often and produces more symptoms in acute renal failure

than in chronic renal failure. In chronic renal failure, compensatory mechanisms maintain acceptable potassium levels. Remaining nephrons filter more potassium, the GI tract increases potassium excretion, and even the skin eliminates some potassium in perspiration.

In acute renal failure, however, these compensatory mechanisms have little opportunity to act because the disorder progresses so quickly. With the rapid deterioration in nephron function, the kidneys can't maintain potassium homeostasis.

Elderly diabetic patients are especially prone to hyperkalemia because their renal function deteriorates as a result of nephron loss and compromised blood flow. Because of chronic illness, these patients typically need medications that further affect nephron integrity. Diabetes likewise decreases the number and function of nephrons. And because insulin promotes cellular uptake of potassium, insufficient endogenous insulin commonly precipitates hyperkalemia.

Assessment findings
When assessing a patient with hyperkalemia, you may detect some or all of these signs and symptoms:
• decreased affect
• nausea
• vomiting
• diarrhea
• hypotension
• bradycardia
• muscle irritability progressing to flaccid paralysis.
Hyperkalemia may also cause cardiac arrest.

Characteristic ECG changes
When the patient has a moderately high serum potassium level (5.5 to 7 mEq/liter), you'll note various ECG changes, such as the following:
• tented T waves (tall, peaked T waves, usually with a narrow base), the earliest sign of hyperkalemia, which develop when the serum potassium level exceeds 5.5 mEq/liter
• flat, broad P waves with decreased amplitude
• prolonged PR interval

Recognizing hyperkalemia

This 12-lead electrocardiogram shows hyperkalemia in a patient with a serum potassium level of 7.5 mEq/liter. Note the characteristic tall, peaked T waves in leads I, II, V_4, V_5, and V_6. Most leads have no P waves or low-amplitude P waves.

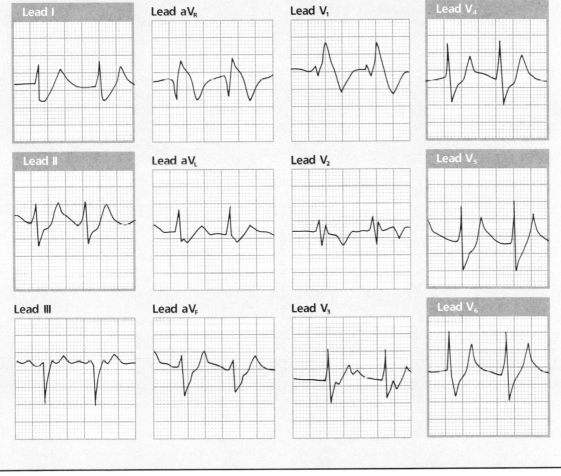

• widened QRS complexes (When the serum potassium level exceeds 6.5 mEq/liter, the QRS complex progressively widens as interventricular conduction slows. A pattern of right or left bundle-branch block may develop.)
• ST-segment depression.
(See *Recognizing hyperkalemia.*)

   With extremely high serum potassium levels (greater than 9 mEq/liter), you may see these ECG changes:
• disappearance of the P wave

• development of sinusoid (sine) waves — wide, bizarre QRS complexes
• ST-segment elevation.

   Other conditions, such as myocardial infarction (MI), may mimic the ECG changes of hyperkalemia. For instance, an acute MI produces an ST-segment elevation, which is easily mistaken for that of severe hyperkalemia. Hyperacute T waves, a hallmark finding in hyperkalemia, also appear as an early sign of ischemia in acute MI, although these T waves tend to be broader and more rounded than those seen in

LEAD OF CHOICE

Monitoring a hyperkalemic patient

When monitoring a patient with hyperkalemia, use lead V_1. With this lead, you can monitor the severity of hyperkalemia by noting the amplitude of the T waves. Also, this lead allows you to quickly detect ventricular arrhythmias, which may develop in a hyperkalemic patient.

Lead V_1   — Tall T waves

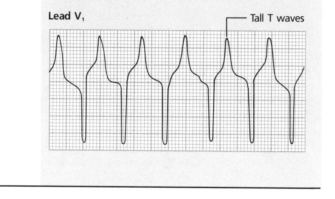

hyperkalemia. What's more, the tall, symmetrical, narrow T waves of hyperkalemia resemble those of an acute posterior MI and are visible from leads V_1 through V_3. Finally, tall, symmetrical T waves may be a normal variation, especially in young athletic males.

Treatment
Therapy aims to correct the underlying cause of hyperkalemia. Cardiac monitoring enhances therapeutic measures by recording ECG changes, allowing you to assess for rhythm and other disturbances. (See *Monitoring a hyperkalemic patient.*)

A dangerously high potassium level may respond to sodium polystyrene sulfonate (Kayexalate) administered orally, rectally, or by nasogastric tube. Other treatments may include an I.V. infusion of sodium bicarbonate or of dextrose and insulin to promote potassium movement into the cell, and administration of diuretics to promote renal excretion of potassium. In a patient with renal failure, dialysis may help remove excess potassium. Emergency

measures for severe hyperkalemia include administering 5 to 10 ml of 10% calcium chloride to protect the myocardium until the potassium level decreases.

After treatment, reassess the patient's serum potassium level every 2 to 4 hours to evaluate the effectiveness of therapy.

Hypokalemia

Changes in myocardial excitability are more complex in hypokalemia than in hyperkalemia. In hypokalemia, the extracellular potassium level falls below 3.5 mEq/liter, and the intracellular potassium level may rise abnormally high. The resulting increase in electrical current across cell membranes enhances excitability and conduction, but only briefly.

After an initial increase in the resting membrane potential, phase 4 (occurring in the Purkinje fibers) lengthens, triggering spontaneous ectopic impulses as the resting maximal diastolic potential decreases. Eventually, the myocardial fibers can't be excited.

Subnormal potassium levels typically result from aldosteronism or Cushing's syndrome (marked by hypersecretion of adrenal steroid hormones), body fluid loss (common in long-term diuretic therapy or extensive burns), or metabolic alkalosis (a possible result of excessive vomiting or gastric suctioning). Dehydration, dieting, malnutrition, and surgery are also possible causes, as are other electrolyte disturbances, such as hypomagnesemia, hypocalcemia, and hyponatremia.

Assessment findings
When assessing a patient with hypokalemia, you may detect some or all of these signs and symptoms:
• fatigue
• lethargy
• apathy
• weak pulse
• tachycardia
• muscle weakness
• respiratory fatigue.

Recognizing hypokalemia

This 12-lead electrocardiogram shows the characteristic changes caused by hypokalemia. Note the prolonged QT interval, caused by prominent U waves, and the decreased T-wave amplitude.

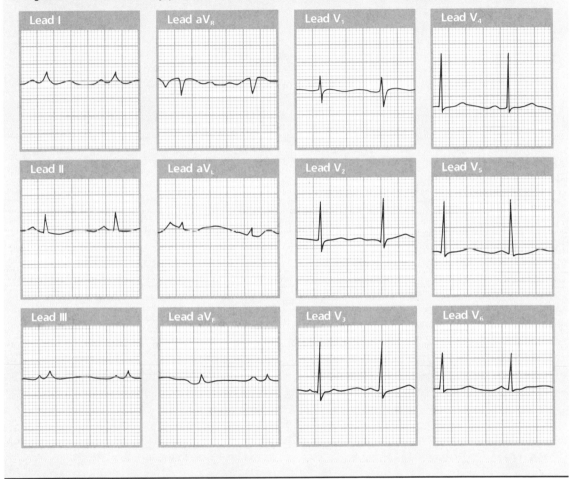

If the patient's serum potassium level decreases further (to less than 2 mEq/liter), he may experience:
• paralytic ileus, possibly progressing to bowel perforation
• ventricular fibrillation
• respiratory paralysis
• cardiac arrest.

Characteristic ECG changes
The ECG changes seen in hypokalemia result from a lengthening of phase 4 of the ventricular action potential. When a patient has hypokalemia, you may see these ECG changes:
• prominent U wave (a hallmark of hypokalemia, occurring in most patients having a serum potassium level less than 2.7 mEq/liter). Low-voltage U waves also become prominent as the serum potassium level falls.
• prolonged PR interval
• ST-segment depression
• decreased T-wave amplitude. As the serum potassium level drops (to under 3 mEq/liter), the T wave flattens. The U wave begins to en-

croach on, then fuse with, the T wave. As hypokalemia progresses, you may see an inverted T wave.
• increased ventricular ectopy.
(See *Recognizing hypokalemia*, page 159, and *Distinguishing between mild and severe hypokalemia*.)

Treatment
Most patients with mild hypokalemia benefit from oral potassium chloride replacement and increased dietary intake. If the patient has a serum potassium level under 3 mEq/liter, he may require I.V. potassium, infused into a central line no faster than 20 mEq/hour.

During the infusion, assess the patient's serum potassium level frequently. Other care measures include performing cardiac monitoring to detect arrhythmias; measuring urine, gastric, fecal, and drainage device output to estimate potassium losses; auscultating bowel sounds to identify possible ileus; and assessing muscle strength and respiratory function.

If the patient is taking digoxin, monitor him carefully and frequently. Digoxin can become toxic even at therapeutic levels in the presence of hypokalemia. Digoxin and potassium compete for the same binding sites on the sodium-potassium pump. With fewer potassium ions available to bind, digoxin levels increase inside the cell.

Calcium imbalances

Bones and teeth store more than 98% of the body's calcium; the extracellular compartment contains the rest. Of the extracellular calcium, about 50% binds to plasma proteins; 10% combines with phosphate, sulfate, and citrate; and the remaining 40% is ionized. Calcium ions play a major role in muscle contraction, normal conduction velocity, excitability, and threshold potential.

Influenced by dietary intake, urine output, GI absorption, and endocrine hormones (which regulate the amount of calcium in bone), serum calcium levels normally range between 4 and 5 mEq/liter. When the ionized calcium level decreases, the parathyroid glands release parathyroid hormone, which stimulates bone to release calcium and the kidneys to reabsorb more calcium.

Calcium levels vary inversely with phosphate levels: When serum calcium levels rise, phosphate levels decrease as a result of renal excretion. Calcium reabsorption in the GI tract depends on sufficient levels of vitamin D. This vitamin is activated in the kidneys, which explains why hypocalcemia commonly accompanies chronic renal failure.

Calcium plays a vital role in the excitation-contraction coupling process in muscle cells. During phase 2 (the plateau phase) of the action potential, calcium enters the cell through slow calcium channels. This calcium prolongs the refractory period and prevents the cell from responding to another impulse. At the same time, calcium ions stimulate the sarcoplasmic reticulum to release more calcium. These calcium ions combine with troponin (a muscle-protein complex), which allows actin and myosin fibers to unite. Cross-bridges form and facilitate muscle contraction.

Hypercalcemia

A patient with hypercalcemia has a serum calcium level greater than 5 mEq/liter. This imbalance may result from Paget's disease, multiple myeloma, metastatic cancer, multiple fractures, prolonged immobilization, or hyperparathyroidism (caused by oversecretion of parathyroid hormone). An elevated serum calcium level may also result from inadequate excretion of calcium, as occurs with adrenal insufficiency and renal disease; from excessive calcium ingestion; or from overuse of antacids containing calcium carbonate.

Assessment findings
When assessing a patient with untreated, severe hypercalcemia, you may detect some or all of these signs and symptoms:
• abdominal pain
• nausea
• vomiting
• constipation

Distinguishing between mild and severe hypokalemia

As serum potassium levels fall, electrocardiogram tracings will change. The following waveforms show changes characteristic of worsening hypokalemia.

Mild hypokalemia
When the serum potassium level slides to 3 mEq/ liter, the T wave and U wave merge, forming a continuous, undulating wave that appears in this view from lead V_2.

Lead V_2

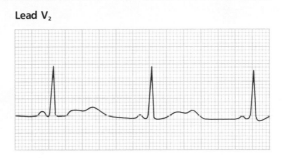

Severe hypokalemia
As the serum potassium level falls to 1.8 mEq/liter, the U wave starts rising above the T wave. Note the characteristic ST-segment depression with prominent U waves in this rhythm strip from lead V_3.

Lead V_3

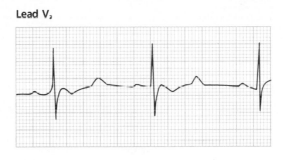

• decreased affect
• confusion
• stupor
• coma
• bone pain (in patients with bone cancer).

Characteristic ECG changes
Hypercalcemia typically produces only subtle ECG changes, if any. However, you may note the following:
• shortened QT interval
• shortened ST segment
• slightly prolonged QRS complex.

Hypercalcemia decreases cell excitability and makes conduction block more likely. It also may potentiate digitalis-induced arrhythmias. (See *Recognizing hypercalcemia,* page 162.)

Treatment
High calcium levels may be diluted with I.V. fluids and lowered with administration of loop diuretics, which promote renal excretion. If the patient doesn't have renal failure, phosphorus may be given orally to promote bone reabsorption of calcium.

The patient with hypercalcemia resulting from metastatic cancer may receive plicamycin, a cytotoxic agent that retards calcium release from bone. The usual dosage is 25 to 30 mcg/ kg/day for 8 to 10 days or until the patient show signs of toxicity, such as bleeding, thrombocytopenia, hepatic and renal impairment, and GI distress.

After giving the patient a test dose to assess hypersensitivity, the doctor may order calcitonin therapy. This hormone inhibits parathyroid hormone activity. If the patient can safely

Recognizing hypercalcemia

This 12-lead electrocardiogram shows the characteristic changes associated with hypercalcemia in a patient with a serum calcium level of 5.6 mEq/liter. Hypercalcemia is indicated by the shortening of the QT interval, primarily due to the shortening of the ST segment.

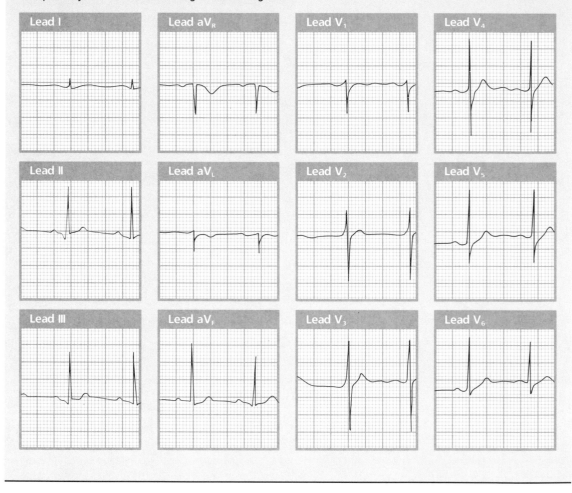

take the usual dosage, you'll administer 4 units/kg, subcutaneously or I.M., every 12 hours.

Hypocalcemia

In hypocalcemia, the patient's low serum calcium level (less than 4 mEq/liter) may result from chronic renal failure, pancreatitis, hypoparathyroidism, dietary inadequacies, or alcoholism. Certain medications — including diuretics, aminoglycosides, estrogen, calcitonin, and adrenocorticosteroids — may also lead to hypocalcemia.

Assessment findings
When assessing a hypocalcemic patient, you may detect some or all of these signs and symptoms:
- numbness and tingling of hands and feet
- twitching

Recognizing hypocalcemia

This 12-lead electrocardiogram shows the characteristic changes associated with hypocalcemia in a patient with a serum calcium level of 3.7 mEq/liter. Hypocalcemia is indicated by a prolonged QT interval. The PR and QRS-complex intervals are within normal limits.

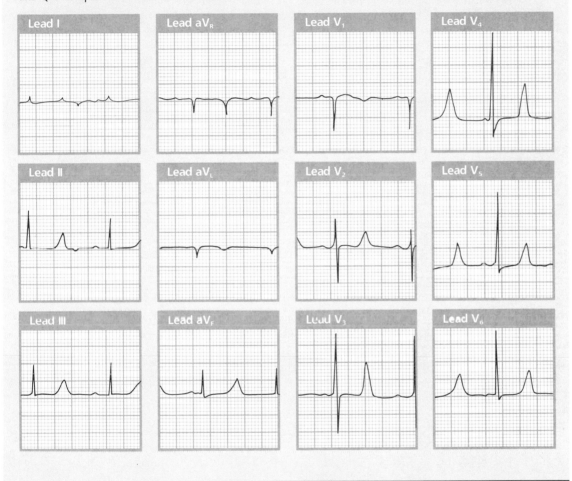

- spasms
- seizures
- tetany.

Characteristic ECG changes
When a patient has hypocalcemia, you may observe these ECG changes:
- prolonged ST segment (the length of the ST segment may be proportional to the decrease in calcium level)
- prolonged QT interval (secondary to ST-segment changes)
- normal T-wave duration, although the T wave may appear somewhat flattened.

Hypocalcemia rarely causes arrhythmias unless the patient also has hypokalemia. (See *Recognizing hypocalcemia.*)

Treatment
For calcium deficiency, treatment includes administering oral calcium and vitamin D supple-

ments. If indicated, the patient may be given 5 to 10 ml of 10% calcium chloride or calcium gluconate (500 to 1,000 mg), administered I.V. no faster than 0.5 ml/minute. If your patient undergoes this treatment, watch for calcium extravasation, which causes tissue necrosis.

If the patient has chronic renal failure, he may receive cholecalciferol, a synthetic form of vitamin D.

Also, continue to assess for symptoms such as tetany, muscle spasms, twitching, and seizures.

Magnesium imbalances

An average-sized adult has total magnesium stores of about 25 g. Normally, bone contains about 60% of the body's magnesium, intracellular fluid holds about 39%, and extracellular structures account for about 1%. The intracellular concentration of magnesium is about 40 mEq/liter, and the extracellular concentration is about 2 mEq/liter. About 30% of extracellular magnesium is bound to plasma proteins or combined with salts, such as phosphate and sulfate. The remaining 70% is ionized and plays an important role in physiologic functions. The normal serum level ranges between 1.5 and 2.5 mEq/liter.

Magnesium, like potassium, is regulated by the kidneys. A healthy adult usually requires 300 to 400 mg of magnesium daily; requirements increase during illness. Whereas the small intestine absorbs about 30% of daily ingested magnesium, the kidneys reabsorb about 95%. When a person ingests too little magnesium, however, the kidneys will reabsorb up to 99%. This increased reabsorption is stimulated partly by parathyroid hormone. Despite this mechanism, some magnesium is lost daily. Persistent magnesium deficiency leads to hypomagnesemia.

Magnesium plays a primary role in the production and use of adenosine triphosphate (ATP), the energy source for most metabolic functions. The body needs magnesium to metabolize glucose, fats, proteins, and nucleic acids. ATP and, thus, magnesium are necessary for chemical reactions at neuromuscular junctions and at various membrane transport systems (for example, the sodium-potassium pump responsible for repolarization in the muscle cells and the sodium-hydrogen pump in the kidneys).

Magnesium influences myocardial cell function in several ways. Because ATP is necessary for the interaction of actin and myosin, magnesium levels affect myocardial contraction. Magnesium also affects myocardial cell excitability by altering the action potential. Dangerously low magnesium levels promote increasing negativity in the resting membrane potential, making the muscle cells more excitable and, possibly, triggering arrhythmias.

Hypermagnesemia

In hypermagnesemia, the patient's serum magnesium level rises above 2.5 mEq/liter. A rare condition, hypermagnesemia usually results from overuse of magnesium-containing antacids, excessive magnesium replacement, dehydration, or chronic renal failure. In chronic renal failure, the renal tubules can't adequately eliminate magnesium, and dialysis may be ineffective.

Assessment findings
Usually, hypermagnesemic patients don't have symptoms until the serum magnesium level exceeds 4 mEq/liter. When assessing a patient with moderate to severe hypermagnesemia, you may detect some or all of these signs and symptoms:
• muscle weakness
• diminished reflexes
• dysphagia
• respiratory depression
• hypotension
• warm, flushed skin
• respiratory and cardiac arrest.

Characteristic ECG changes
Initially, you may see slight ECG changes in a patient with hypermagnesemia. If the magnesium levels continue to rise, the ECG changes will intensify. These changes include:

Recognizing hypermagnesemia

This 12-lead electrocardiogram shows the characteristic changes associated with hypermagnesemia in a patient with a magnesium level of 4.2 mEq/liter. Note the prolonged PR intervals, wide QRS complexes, and tall T waves.

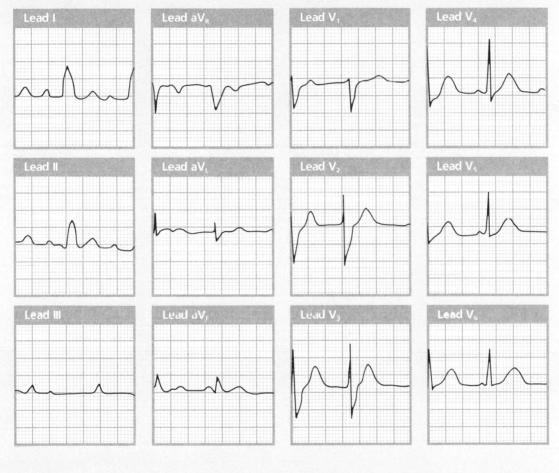

- prolonged PR interval
- widened QRS complex
- tall T wave
- atrioventricular block.
(See *Recognizing hypermagnesemia.*)

Treatment
Immediate treatment for hypermagnesemia involves stopping all magnesium supplements and, in cases of severe hypermagnesemia, ad-

ministering 5 to 10 ml of 10% calcium gluconate solution. The patient may also require hemodialysis or peritoneal dialysis to remove excess magnesium from the body.

Hypomagnesemia

In hypomagnesemia, the serum magnesium level falls below 1.5 mEq/liter. Unfortunately, serum magnesium levels don't accurately re-

Recognizing hypomagnesemia

This 12-lead electrocardiogram shows the changes caused by a magnesium level of 0.91 mEq/liter. Note the tall T waves in most of the leads. The duration of the QT interval is prolonged.

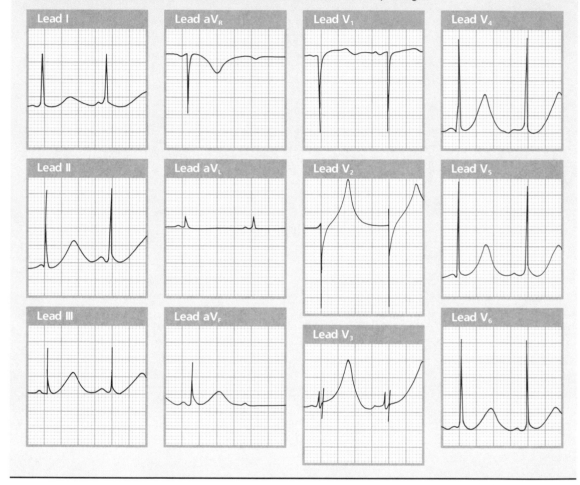

flect intracellular magnesium levels. A patient may have a low, normal, or slightly elevated serum magnesium level, yet be intracellularly depleted. Because intracellular magnesium levels are difficult to measure, they aren't routinely evaluated.

About 10% of hospitalized patients have magnesium deficiencies; the incidence may be as high as 60% in critically ill patients. Among hospitalized patients, the causes of hypomagnesemia include sepsis, excessive catecholamine release, various medications, excessive body

fluid losses, and inadequate replacement therapy. Within the first 16 hours after an MI, many patients experience transient hypomagnesemia related to catecholamine release.

Magnesium deficiency usually results from large losses of magnesium in the urine or feces. In some disorders, such as glomerulonephritis and acute renal failure, the kidneys fail to conserve magnesium adequately. The same situation results from diuretic therapy, hyperaldosteronism, hypercalcemia, and hyperparathyroidism. As well, various hormones and medications increase renal excretion of magnesium. Nutritional deficits aren't generally thought to cause magnesium deficiency, although increased consumption of processed foods, which may be magnesium deficient, may result in borderline hypomagnesemia.

Hypomagnesemia is typically associated with hypokalemia, hypocalcemia, and hypophosphatemia. These associations stem from the sodium-potassium pump's dependence on magnesium to function properly. For example, a patient with hypomagnesemia will also experience hypokalemia because his body needs adequate magnesium to promote potassium reabsorption.

Assessment findings

When assessing a patient who has hypomagnesemia, you may detect some or all of these signs and symptoms:
• ventricular arrhythmias
• neuromuscular irritability
• hyperactive reflexes
• altered level of consciousness.

Characteristic ECG changes

The ECG changes that suggest hypomagnesemia are thought to stem from magnesium's role in regulating the sodium-potassium pump and, thus, its effect on the resting membrane potential and repolarization.

When a patient has chronic magnesium deficiency, you may see the following ECG changes:
• slightly prolonged PR interval
• slightly prolonged QRS complex
• ST-segment depression
• broad, flattened T waves
• prominent U waves
• prolonged QT interval.

When the magnesium level falls below 1.1 mEq/liter, you may see the following ECG changes:
• narrowed QRS complex
• tall, peaked T waves.

When the magnesium level falls below 0.85 mEq/liter and is accompanied by increased ventricular ectopy, you may see the following ECG changes:

• ventricular tachycardia
• ventricular fibrillation
• torsades de pointes, possibly caused by afterdepolarization.
(See *Recognizing hypomagnesemia.*)

Treatment

If pulseless ventricular tachycardia, ventricular fibrillation, and torsades de pointes accompany hypomagnesemia, emergency treatment calls for I.V. magnesium replacement (1 to 2 g infused over several minutes). If the patient has stable ventricular tachycardia, magnesium should be infused over 15 to 30 minutes to decrease the risk of hypotension triggered by administering the magnesium too fast.

Because cellular uptake of magnesium occurs gradually and because the kidneys excrete most of the initial magnesium dose, the patient will need follow-up doses (typically, 1 g I.V. every 8 hours for 3 days). Other treatment measures include performing continuous cardiac monitoring, assessing magnesium levels daily to detect hypermagnesemia and, if indicated, administering calcium as a magnesium antagonist.

PART 4

Understanding the effects of treatment

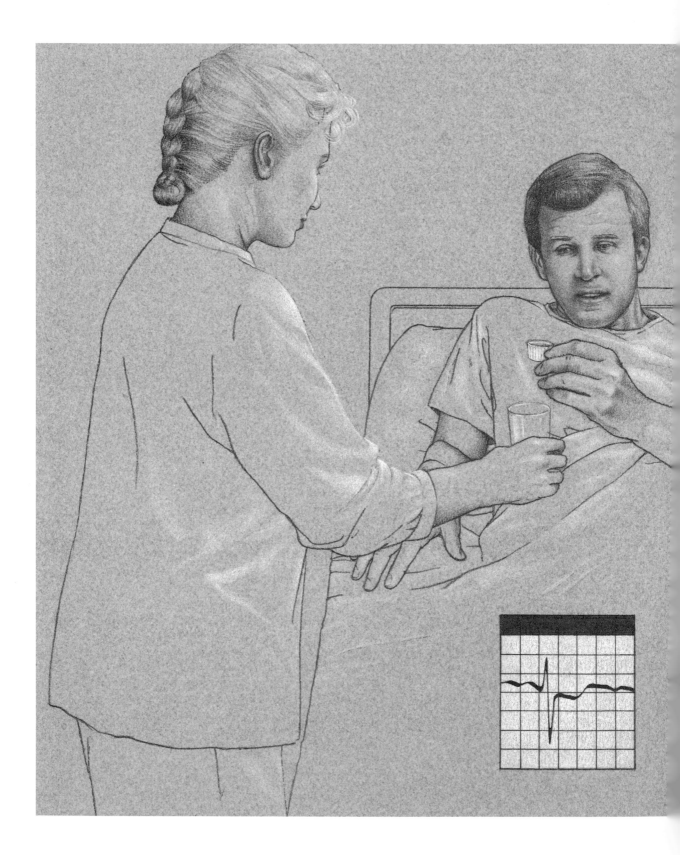

CHAPTER 12

Antiarrhythmic drugs

Each year in North America, more than 400,000 people die suddenly from cardiac arrhythmias. Plus, countless others suffer from conditions brought on by arrhythmias. Although surgery and permanent implanted pacemakers are now used to treat some affected patients, antiarrhythmic drugs remain the mainstay of therapy for most.

More than two dozen antiarrhythmics are now available, and each one has the potential to be not only lifesaving but also life-threatening. In some patients, antiarrhythmic drugs can worsen existing arrhythmias or trigger new ones. That's why you must monitor your patient closely after giving an antiarrhythmic. And your primary monitoring tool is the electrocardiogram (ECG). In effect, the ECG can provide early warning of drug-induced complications so prompt intervention can begin.

In this chapter, you'll find an overview of antiarrhythmics that explains how they can worsen existing arrhythmias and cause new ones. You'll also find information about specific drugs in each class of antiarrhythmics. For each drug, you'll find its effect on the action potential, its indications and recommended dosage, characteristic ECG changes, and nursing considerations for administration and monitoring.

Understanding antiarrhythmics

A pharmacologically diverse group of drugs, antiarrhythmics do share one common feature: They alter the flow of ionic currents across the cell membrane, thus altering the heart's electrophysiology. Depending on their electrophysiologic effects, the antiarrhythmic drugs are grouped into four classes, with class I further divided into three subclasses:
• Class I drugs block the fast influx of sodium. Drugs in class IA prolong the action potential and moderately reduce conductivity. In contrast, drugs in class IB shorten repolarization and the refractory period and cause little or no change in conductivity. Drugs in class IC markedly reduce conduction.
• Class II drugs block beta-adrenergic receptors.
• Class III drugs block potassium channels and prolong repolarization and the refractory period.
• Class IV drugs block calcium channels.

This classification scheme has some limitations, however. Although it predicts the ECG features of the antiarrhythmics, many of the drugs don't fit neatly into just one class. Some produce effects typical of several classes. For example, amiodarone is considered a member of class III, but some of its effects are more typical of class I, II, and IV drugs.

Plus, some antiarrhythmic drugs produce metabolites that have different actions than the parent drug. A case in point: Procainamide, a class IA drug, blocks sodium channels. But its major metabolite, N-acetylprocainamide, exerts only class III action; that is, it prolongs repolarization. The effects of procainamide depend on the concentration of this metabolite, which in

turn depends on the presence of the hepatic enzyme N-acetyltransferase. The activity of this enzyme varies markedly among patients.

Despite these limitations, though, the classification scheme remains useful for understanding the different types of antiarrhythmics and their effects on the ECG. That's because each of the four classes affects a different phase of the action potential. (See *Antiarrhythmics and the action potential*.)

Drug distribution and clearance

When you infuse an antiarrhythmic, blood levels will initially be high in well-perfused organs, such as the heart, liver, and kidneys. Then, as the drug is distributed throughout the rest of the body, its concentration in these organs will diminish. This may explain why drug-induced arrhythmias are more likely to occur early in treatment, when cardiac concentrations are high. With time, as cardiac concentrations diminish, the risk of toxicity and drug-induced arrhythmias also declines.

Most antiarrhythmics are cleared by the liver and the kidneys. As a result, altered blood flow to these organs can affect drug clearance—and heighten the risk of toxicity. Such alteration can stem from low cardiac output, compromised renal function, and concurrent use of drugs that induce hepatic enzymes.

Proarrhythmias

All antiarrhythmic drugs can be proarrhythmic—that is, they can cause or exacerbate arrhythmias. Arrhythmias caused or worsened by drugs (or other therapy) have come to be known as *proarrhythmias*. Proarrhythmias include sustained ventricular tachycardia, ventricular fibrillation, torsades de pointes, and ventricular standstill. Proarrhythmias can cause transient ischemic attacks, heart failure, angina, myocardial infarction, (MI), and sudden death. (See *Depicting proarrhythmias on the action potential curve*, page 174.)

Antiarrhythmics and the action potential

Each class of antiarrhythmic drugs acts on a different phase of the cardiac action potential to alter the heart's electrophysiology.

Class I drugs
These sodium channel blockers reduce the influx of sodium ions during phase 0 of the action potential.

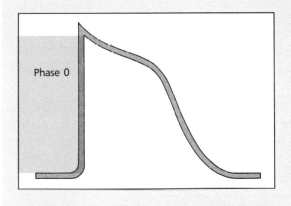

Class II drugs
These drugs inhibit adrenergic stimulation of cardiac tissue. They depress phase 4 depolarization and slow sinoatrial (SA) node impulses.

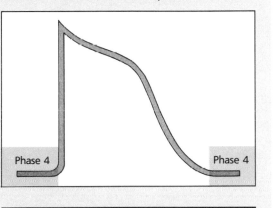

Class III drugs
These potassium channel blockers prolong phase 3 of the action potential, thereby increasing repolarization and refractoriness.

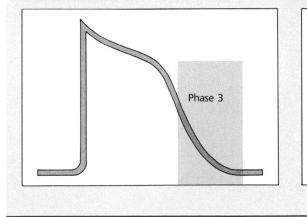

Class IV drugs
These drugs inhibit calcium's slow influx during the action potential's plateau phase (phase 2). They depress phase 4 and lengthen phases 1 and 2.

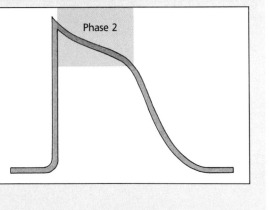

Risk factors
Although the exact mechanisms that trigger proarrhythmias are unknown, certain factors predispose patients to them. Major ones include fluid and electrolyte imbalances and structural damage to the myocardium—particularly ischemic tissue injury.

When a patient has an electrolyte imbalance, changes in pH and circulating levels of catecholamines may amplify the proarrhythmic

Depicting proarrhythmias on the action potential curve

How can a single drug treat arrhythmias in some patients—and cause them in others? These two sets of illustrations of the action potential show these opposite effects.

Drug stopping an arrhythmia
The illustration below represents an arrhythmia caused by an ectopic focus discharging during phase 3 of the action potential.

This next illustration shows the action potential after antiarrhythmic treatment has prolonged the refractory period. This stops the premature ectopic discharge, suppressing the arrhythmia.

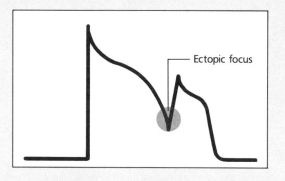

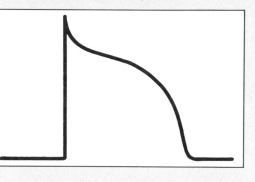

Drug causing an arrhythmia
The illustration below shows a borderline arrhythmia. Here the ectopic focus occurs but discharges normally without drug treatment.

When the antiarrhythmic drug prolongs the refractory period, the ectopic focus discharges in phase 3, promoting a proarrhythmia.

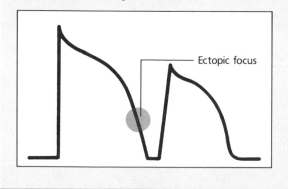

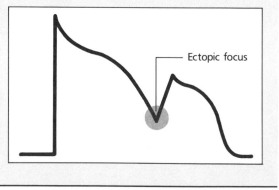

effect of some antiarrhythmic drugs. And in a patient with myocardial ischemia, an antiarrhythmic drug may not only suppress abnormal rhythms that originate in diseased tissue but may also depress healthy tissue. Antiarrhythmics also can change ischemic cells into active foci for abnormal automatic or reentry circuits,

triggering proarrhythmias. (See *How a proarrhythmia develops*.)

When your patient is receiving an antiarrhythmic, be aware of these additional risk factors for proarrhythmias:
• a history of sustained ventricular tachycardia or ventricular fibrillation

• coronary artery disease or significant valvular disease
• severe left ventricular dysfunction
• diuretic therapy with or without electrolyte imbalances
• hypokalemia or hypomagnesemia
• long QT syndrome before antiarrhythmic therapy.

Assessment findings

Because antiarrhythmics have a narrow therapeutic range, you must assess patients carefully before and during therapy. Before therapy, focus on underlying conditions that may increase the patient's risk of developing proarrhythmias and other adverse reactions. Once therapy begins, assess his cardiovascular, respiratory, nervous, and GI systems.

Cardiovascular system
Regularly assess the patient's blood pressure, pulse, and capillary refill. Note if he has hypotension, a common effect of antiarrhythmic therapy. Ask about cardiac symptoms, such as fatigue, activity intolerance, chest pain, and palpitations.

Respiratory system
Assessment of the lungs is important for two reasons. First, many patients with arrhythmias also suffer from respiratory disorders. Second, certain antiarrhythmics can aggravate underlying respiratory diseases. For example, class II drugs are usually contraindicated in patients with asthma because they block beta-adrenergic receptors, which can aggravate bronchospasm.

Several other antiarrhythmics, particularly amiodarone and tocainide, can cause pulmonary fibrosis. If your patient is receiving one of these drugs, regularly evaluate him for dyspnea and a nonproductive cough—the most common symptoms. The doctor also may order periodic chest X-rays, pulmonary function tests, and other studies.

PATHOPHYSIOLOGY

How a proarrhythmia develops

These illustrations show you how an antiarrhythmic drug can cause a borderline arrhythmia to deteriorate into a proarrhythmia.

Borderline arrhythmia
In the illustration below, before antiarrhythmic therapy, notice how conduction is slowed through an ischemic area of muscle fiber. Even so, the impulse continues in antegrade fashion, and no arrhythmia results.

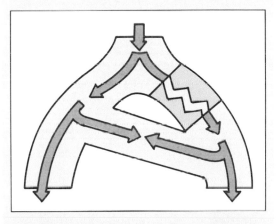

Drug-induced arrhythmia
Now look what happens after antiarrhythmic therapy. In this illustration, conduction through the area of ischemia is even further depressed, triggering the reentry circuit.

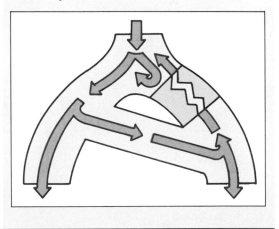

Nervous system

Although neurologic complications generally aren't life-threatening, they can be troublesome and may require dosage adjustment. Although all antiarrhythmics can cause neurologic complications, lidocaine and amiodarone are among the biggest offenders.

During your assessment, ask the patient about neurologic symptoms, such as headache, drowsiness, confusion, tremor, and numbness. Also ask if he has had any difficulty breathing, swallowing, or seeing.

GI system

Antiarrhythmic drugs are well known for producing adverse GI effects. Although such complications usually occur with oral drugs, such as quinidine and mexiletine, they can also arise with I.V. lidocaine.

During your assessment, check for nausea, vomiting, diarrhea, and other signs of GI upset. Because liver damage is commonly associated with long-term antiarrhythmic therapy, the doctor may order periodic liver function tests.

Characteristic ECG changes

Because ECG changes depend on the type of antiarrhythmic, they'll be covered later under the various drug classifications. But keep in mind that even therapeutic doses can cause significant ECG changes. Consequently, during cardiac monitoring, be alert for iatrogenic arrhythmias and try to determine if their configuration signals drug toxicity. Also be alert for bradycardia, which reduces cardiac output and lowers blood pressure.

Class I antiarrhythmics

Also known as membrane-stabilizing agents, these antiarrhythmics are potent local nerve anesthetics that depress the excitability of cardiac muscle.

Class IA antiarrhythmics

This category includes quinidine, procainamide, and disopyramide. These drugs block the sodium channel, decreasing the rate of depolarization and prolonging the duration of the action potential. They delay the return of excitability, lengthening the effective refractory period. Plus, they can inhibit muscarinic receptors to cause an anticholinergic effect.

If your patient is receiving a class IA drug, monitor his ECG closely. Because these drugs prolong the QT interval, they can trigger proarrhythmias, especially ventricular arrhythmias.

Characteristic ECG changes

During class IA antiarrhythmic therapy, you may note the following changes on the ECG:
• increased P-wave duration
• prolonged QT interval
• prominent U wave
• ST-segment depression
• decreased T-wave amplitude
• T-wave inversion.

The drug most commonly associated with these changes is quinidine. (See *Class IA antiarrhythmics: Effects on the ECG.*)

These ECG changes may indicate drug toxicity:
• prolonged QRS complex
• sinus bradycardia
• sinus arrest
• sinoatrial (SA) block
• atrioventricular (AV) block
• torsades de pointes.

Typically, when drug-induced torsades de pointes develops, it does so within a few days of the start of therapy. Examine the patient's ECG for progressive lengthening of the QT interval and a prominent U wave—two of the most important warning signs.

Quinidine

The most widely used antiarrhythmic drug, quinidine effectively treats many supraventricular and ventricular arrhythmias, including atrial flutter and fibrillation and paroxysmal supraventricular tachycardia (SVT). Because quinidine produces a vagolytic effect, blocking conduction along the AV nodal pathway, it's indicated

Class IA antiarrhythmics: Effects on the ECG

This class of antiarrhythmic drugs causes the following electrocardiogram (ECG) changes: a slightly widened QRS complex and a prolonged QT interval.

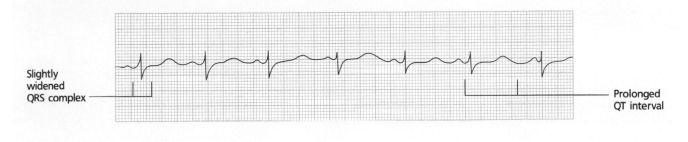

Slightly widened QRS complex

Prolonged QT interval

for reentrant tachycardia in the atrium, AV junction, and ventricles.

Dosage
Typically, you'll administer an initial oral dose of 200 mg to check for hypersensitivity. After this dose, begin sustained oral therapy of 200 to 300 mg every 3 to 4 hours, not to exceed 2 g/day. Long-acting preparations, such as quinidine gluconate and quinidine polygalacturonate, have similar limits.

Characteristic ECG changes
Quinidine produces many electrophysiologic effects, including prolonged ventricular conduction time, repolarization, and refractoriness. When your patient is taking this drug, you may note these changes on his ECG:
• prolonged PR interval
• prolonged QRS complex
• prolonged QT interval.
(See *Recognizing quinidine toxicity,* page 178.)

Nursing considerations
• If your patient is experiencing atrial fibrillation, give digoxin before quinidine, as ordered. Otherwise, a life-threatening ventricular arrhythmia may result.
• Because quinidine can heighten the risk of digoxin toxicity, use the two drugs cautiously. Be sure to monitor digoxin levels.
• Closely monitor changes in the patient's QT

interval and QRS complex, especially when administering the initial dose of quinidine. A prolonged QT interval is associated with ventricular tachycardia or torsades de pointes.
• Because quinidine can cause vasodilation, watch for hypotension, especially if you're giving a high loading dose. Closely monitor a patient receiving an antihypertensive drug.
• Watch for adverse GI reactions, such as nausea, vomiting, and diarrhea. To prevent GI upset, give quinidine with meals. If symptoms develop, provide antacids with aluminum derivatives, as appropriate.

Procainamide
This drug is used to treat many supraventricular and ventricular arrhythmias. It's commonly given intravenously to patients who don't respond to lidocaine.

Dosage and pharmacodynamics
The usual oral regimen is a loading dose of 1 g, followed by 500 mg every 3 to 4 hours. With the slow-release preparation, the usual dose, which is the same as the oral regimen, is given every 6 hours. The I.V. regimen consists of a loading dose of 1 g given over 1 hour and then a maintenance dose of 2 to 6 mg/minute.

Procainamide reaches its peak effect in 1 to 1½ hours, and plateau plasma levels occur in 12 to 24 hours. The therapeutic level ranges

Recognizing quinidine toxicity

Like most antiarrhythmic drugs, quinidine has a narrow therapeutic window. That means you'll need to monitor the patient's electrocardiogram closely, so you can distinguish acceptable electrophysiologic changes from warning signs of quinidine toxicity.

This strip is from a patient with aortic stenosis receiving quinidine because of previous ventricular arrhythmias. Note the regular sinus rhythm (PR interval is 0.20 second). The R wave in lead aV_L is

14 mm. You can also observe ST-segment depression and T-wave inversion in leads I, aV_L, and V_4 through V_6. The R-wave voltage in aV_L and some of the other ST-T changes reflect left ventricular hypertrophy.

Now look at leads V_2 and V_3. The effects of quinidine are clear. Notice the prolonged QT interval (0.60 second). Such marked prolongation indicates drug toxicity.

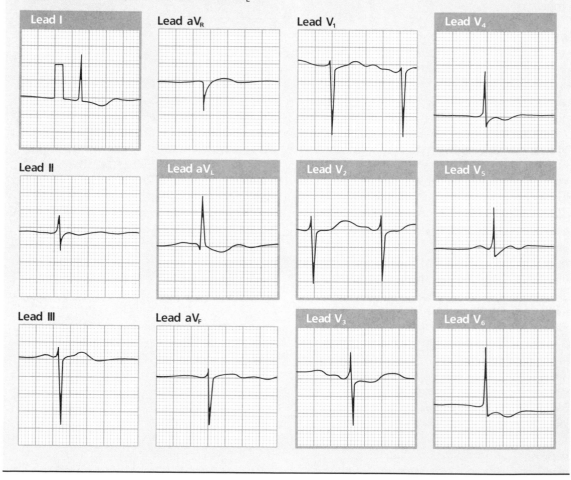

from 4 to 10 mcg/ml. Peak plasma concentration after I.V. administration is 30% higher than after oral administration of the same dose.

In a patient with normal renal function, 50% of the drug is excreted in 3 to 4 hours. In a patient with renal insufficiency or congestive heart failure (CHF), drug elimination will be slower, and the doctor will reduce the dosage.

Characteristic ECG changes

Although procainamide produces effects similar to those of quinidine, the drug is less vagolytic because it has less interaction with muscarinic receptors. The result on an ECG may be enhanced AV conduction, which would increase the ventricular rate in atrial flutter or fibrillation. If your patient is receiving procainamide, you may observe these changes on his ECG:
• prolonged PR interval
• prolonged QRS complex
• minor lengthening of QT interval.

Nursing considerations

• When administering the loading dose, don't let the flow rate exceed 25 mg/minute, or the patient may develop hypotension.
• If the patient is receiving procainamide I.V., monitor his blood pressure and ECG continuously. Watch for a prolonged QT interval and QRS complex, heart block, and worsening arrhythmias. If any of these occur, withhold the drug, obtain a rhythm strip, and notify the doctor immediately.
• If the patient develops "breakthrough" ectopy, you may be ordered to administer extra procainamide. Typically, you'll give a supplemental bolus of 100 to 200 mg over 5 to 10 minutes, followed by an increase in the maintenance dose in increments of 1 mg/minute.
• If the patient is taking a sustained-release oral preparation, inform him that the drug capsule, which is coated with a waxy material, may appear in his stools.
• Monitor the patient's blood urea nitrogen and serum creatinine levels. Remember, the risk of drug toxicity rises with poor renal function.
• Be aware that long-term procainamide treatment isn't recommended because the drug has been linked to the development of lupus erythematosus.

Disopyramide

Typically, disopyramide is ordered when quinidine or procainamide treatment fails. The drug is indicated for premature ventricular contractions (PVCs) and ventricular tachycardia not severe enough to require electrocardioversion. However, disopyramide's usefulness is limited by its negative inotropic and anticholinergic effects.

Dosage and pharmacodynamics

Disopyramide is only given orally. The usual dose is 300 mg initially, followed by 100 to 200 mg every 6 hours. You'll administer long-acting preparations, such as Norpace CR and Rythmodan-LA, every 12 hours.

About 90% of the drug is absorbed, with the peak plasma levels occurring after 6 to 8 hours in patients with good renal function. Disopyramide is mainly eliminated through the kidneys, with some metabolism in the liver. The drug has a long half-life (13 to 107 days) and elimination period (12 months). It accumulates progressively in the tissues, reaching peak concentrations in 1 to 3 weeks.

Characteristic ECG changes

Generally, disopyramide has the same effects on the ECG as quinidine and procainamide. However, because disopyramide possesses more of an anticholinergic effect than quinidine, it may cause rebound sympathetic stimulation. Therefore, you may observe a slight increase in heart rate.

Nursing considerations

• In patients with CHF, use disopyramide cautiously or avoid it altogether. The risk of heart failure may be increased in these patients because disopyramide has a greater negative inotropic effect than quinidine or procainamide.
• Because this drug inhibits muscarinic receptors, watch for anticholinergic effects, such as urine retention, worsening of glaucoma, and constipation.
• Carefully monitor the patient's ECG, paying close attention to changes in the QRS complex and the QT interval. Discontinue the drug, as ordered, if heart block develops, if the QRS complex widens by more than 25%, or if the QT interval lengthens by more than 25% from baseline.

Class IB antiarrhythmics: Effects on the ECG

These drugs produce the following electrocardiogram (ECG) changes: a shortened or slightly prolonged PR interval and a slightly widened QRS complex.

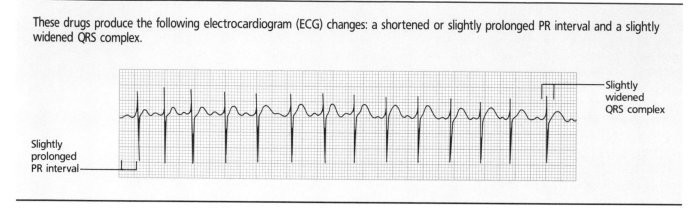

Slightly prolonged PR interval

Slightly widened QRS complex

Class IB antiarrhythmics

This group of drugs includes lidocaine, mexiletine, tocainide, moricizine, and phenytoin. Class IB drugs depress phase 0 slightly and shorten the action potential. They produce a stronger effect on ischemic myocardial tissue than on healthy tissue. As a result, they help to promote conduction block, thereby interrupting a reentry circuit.

Class IB antiarrhythmics are used to treat ventricular automaticity and arrhythmias. With the exception of moricizine, these drugs aren't effective against atrial arrhythmias.

Characteristic ECG changes
Because class IB drugs have a negligible effect on depolarization or repolarization, they cause few changes on the ECG. Usually, they produce little change in the PR interval and QRS complex, although occasionally you may note a shortened PR or QT interval. (See *Class IB antiarrhythmics: Effects on the ECG.*)

Lidocaine
Because of its affinity for ischemic myocardial tissue, lidocaine is the drug of choice for suppressing ventricular arrhythmias.

Dosage and pharmacodynamics
Typically, you'll administer a loading dose of 75 mg I.V., followed by two to three 50-mg

boluses at 5-minute intervals. The total loading dose is 100 to 200 mg I.V. or 400 mg I.M.

Lidocaine is rapidly distributed after the initial loading dose. So start a continuous drip at 2 to 4 mg/minute as soon as you've given the loading dose.

Lidocaine's therapeutic plasma level is reached 5 to 9 hours after starting a continuous infusion. The drug is effectively eliminated by the liver.

Nursing considerations
• While the patient is receiving a continuous lidocaine infusion, watch for breakthrough ventricular arrhythmias—short runs of ventricular tachycardia. If they occur, the doctor may order a supplemental I.V. bolus of 25 to 50 mg, then increase the maintenance infusion by 1 mg/minute.
• Be aware that altered hepatic blood flow can interfere with lidocaine elimination. Watch for signs of toxicity in patients who have CHF, decreased cardiac output, or cirrhosis. Signs of toxicity include confusion, dizziness, hallucinations, paresthesia and, in extreme toxicity, seizures and coma. If toxic signs develop, stop the drug at once and notify the doctor.

Mexiletine
Similar in structure and action to lidocaine, mexiletine has one important distinction: It can be given orally because it's well absorbed from

the GI tract. The drug's main indication is treatment of refractory ventricular arrhythmias.

Dosage and pharmacodynamics
If a high initial level is needed, you'll usually administer an oral loading dose of 400 mg. Two to six hours later, you'll give 300 to 1,200 mg in three divided doses. Long-acting preparations contain 360 mg and should be given twice a day.

Peak plasma levels occur in 2 to 4 hours. Therapeutic levels range from 0.75 to 2 mg/ml. The drug is metabolized in the liver.

Nursing considerations
• To minimize gastric irritation, give mexiletine after meals or with an antacid. Because the drug is largely absorbed after gastric digestion, delayed gastric emptying may alter plasma concentrations.
• To avoid possible drug interactions, use the drug cautiously in patients who are also receiving narcotics, hepatic enzyme inducers (alcohol, phenytoin, phenobarbital, rifampin), disopyramide, beta blockers, or cimetidine. Also, theophylline and caffeine may increase mexiletine levels and the risk of tachyarrhythmias.
• Use caution when giving I.V. lidocaine concurrently with mexiletine because of the risk of additive central nervous system (CNS) effects.
• This drug has a narrow therapeutic range. As a result, fewer than 25% of patients sustain the antiarrhythmic effect without experiencing significant adverse reactions. Assess your patient for toxic signs and symptoms, such as tremor, dizziness, ataxia, and nystagmus.

Tocainide
Considered an "oral lidocaine," tocainide has a similar structure and actions. Its main indication is the suppression of symptomatic ventricular arrhythmias, including frequent PVCs and ventricular tachycardia.

The doctor may order tocainide to ease the transition from I.V. lidocaine to oral antiarrhythmic therapy. Tocainide has a minimal negative inotropic effect on the myocardium.

Dosage
The usual oral dosage is 300 to 600 mg two to three times a day.

Nursing considerations
• Use the drug cautiously in patients with compromised pulmonary function because the drug can cause pulmonary fibrosis.
• Monitor the patient for signs and symptoms of CNS or GI toxicity: paresthesia, dizziness, light-headedness, nausea, tremor, and vomiting. Give the drug with food.
• Monitor the patient for easy bleeding or bruising. Tocainide can inhibit coagulation.

Moricizine
A phenothiazine derivative, moricizine differs from other class IB drugs in that it suppresses both atrial and ventricular arrhythmias. The drug treats life-threatening ventricular arrhythmias and supraventricular arrhythmias. It's usually well tolerated.

Dosage and pharmacodynamics
Typically, you'll administer an oral dose of 600 to 900 mg, divided in three doses at 8-hour intervals.

Moricizine is predominantly metabolized in the liver. The drug's half-life is 2 to 5 hours, which may be prolonged in patients with renal insufficiency.

Nursing considerations
• Give moricizine with meals.
• Monitor the patient for proarrhythmias, especially during the first week of therapy.

Phenytoin
Although phenytoin isn't approved as an antiarrhythmic, it's commonly prescribed to treat arrhythmias induced by digoxin. It's also used to treat ventricular arrhythmias that are unresponsive to lidocaine or procainamide.

Dosage and pharmacodynamics
The recommended regimen is 10 to 15 mg/kg I.V. administered over 1 hour, followed by an oral maintenance dosage of 400 to 600 mg/day.

Phenytoin is absorbed mainly through the

GI tract. Its peak effect occurs in 3 to 9 hours, with plateau plasma levels in 6 to 7 days. The therapeutic plasma level is 10 to 18 mcg/ml.

Because phenytoin is metabolized primarily in the liver, it can affect hepatic enzymes. As a result, the doctor may order dosage adjustments in other antiarrhythmic drugs.

Nursing considerations
• Because phenytoin solution is highly alkaline, administer it through a central line to prevent phlebitis. Also, to prevent precipitation in the line, dissolve the phenytoin in 0.9% sodium chloride solution and infuse it without glucose.
• Administer the I.V. loading dose slowly to prevent hypotension.
• To prevent gingival hyperplasia, explain the need for proper oral hygiene and regular dental examinations.

Class IC antiarrhythmics

Drugs in this category—flecainide, encainide, and propafenone—inhibit the sodium channel and depress phase 0. Although these drugs slow conduction profoundly, they affect repolarization only slightly. They differ from class IA and class IB drugs in that they do not prolong or shorten the action potential.

Class IC drugs are potent antiarrhythmics. However, serious doubts concerning their safety have recently come to light. Because class IC drugs often exhibit proarrhythmic effects, they are now restricted for use only in patients with life-threatening ventricular arrhythmias.

Characteristic ECG changes
When your patient is receiving a class IC antiarrhythmic, you may note the following changes on his ECG:
• prolonged PR interval
• widened QRS complex
• prolonged QT interval.

Class IC drugs inhibit conduction in the His-Purkinje network, causing a widening of the QRS complex. Excessive widening may indicate an overdose. The increase in the QT interval primarily reflects the widening of the QRS complex. (See *Class IC antiarrhythmics: Effects on the ECG.*)

Flecainide
The first class IC antiarrhythmic to be developed, flecainide is now used only to treat life-threatening ventricular arrhythmias, such as ventricular tachycardia.

Dosage and pharmacodynamics
Usually, you'll give flecainide in oral doses of 100 to 400 mg twice daily.

After oral administration, flecainide is rapidly and completely absorbed from the GI tract. The drug is metabolized in the liver and has a half-life of 20 hours.

Nursing considerations
• Be aware that drug interactions may occur in patients taking beta blockers, verapamil, diltiazem, or digitalis.
• Because flecainide depresses myocardial contractility, use it cautiously (if at all) in patients with myocardial ischemia accompanied by ventricular dysfunction.
• Instruct the patient not to take flecainide with meals. Food ingestion delays, but does not reduce, drug absorption.

Encainide
This drug was voluntarily withdrawn from the market by the manufacturer in 1991. However, because some doctors are reluctant to switch their patients to another antiarrhythmic agent, encainide is still available on a limited basis for patients whose arrhythmias are effectively controlled by it.

Dosage
The usual dosage of encainide is 25 to 75 mg P.O., three times daily.

Nursing considerations
• If the patient is taking cimetidine, use encainide cautiously. Cimetidine may increase encainide blood levels.
• Because encainide is metabolized primarily in the liver, hepatic enzyme inducers may decrease its blood levels.
• Monitor the patient for new or worsened ar-

Class IC antiarrhythmics: Effects on the ECG

These drugs produce the following electrocardiogram (ECG) changes: a prolonged PR interval, a widened QRS complex, and a prolonged QT interval.

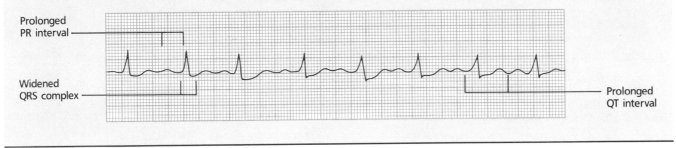

rhythmias. Proarrhythmic events usually occur during the first week of therapy and are more common at higher doses.

Propafenone
Propafenone is used only for life-threatening ventricular arrhythmias.

Dosage
Approved only for oral administration, propafenone is usually given in doses of 150 to 300 mg three times daily. The maximum daily dose is 1,200 mg.

Nursing considerations
• Use this drug cautiously in patients taking digitalis. Propafenone can increase serum digoxin levels, potentially causing a depressant effect on the conduction system.
• Monitor patients receiving warfarin for easy bruising and bleeding because propafenone can increase warfarin's plasma concentration.

Class II antiarrhythmics

Also known as beta-adrenergic blockers, these drugs treat supraventricular and ventricular arrhythmias. They also help to prevent pacemaker-induced atrial and ventricular tachycardia.

Beta blockers are most useful when the arrhythmia stems from excessive catecholamine levels, as with myocardial ischemia. They may also be used to treat arrhythmias of mitral valve prolapse.

Because these drugs prevent the influx of calcium ions, they have a negative inotropic effect. By lowering cytoplasmic calcium levels, they reduce the peak force of myocardial contractions.

Types of class II antiarrhythmics

Beta blockers act by blocking beta receptors, of which there are two types: beta-1 receptors, found primarily in cardiac tissue, and beta-2 receptors, found in bronchial and vascular smooth muscle. Blocking beta-1 receptors reduces heart rate, conduction, and contractility. Blocking beta-2 receptors results in smooth muscle contraction and bronchospasm.

Class II antiarrhythmics are subdivided into three groups, based on the type of beta receptor they block:
• Nonselective beta blockers obstruct beta-1 and beta-2 receptors. These drugs include nadolol, oxprenolol, propranolol, sotalol, and timolol.
• Cardioselective beta blockers obstruct beta-1

Dosages for class II antiarrhythmics

DRUG	USUAL DOSAGE
Nonselective beta blockers	
Nadolol (Corgard)	Oral: 80 to 240 mg once a day; mean dose is 100 mg
Oxprenolol (Trasicor)	Oral: 120 to 140 mg/day (t.i.d. or q.i.d.) I.V.: 1 to 12 mg
Propranolol (Inderal) (Inderal LA)	Oral: 120 to 140 mg/day (t.i.d. or q.i.d.) I.V.: 0.1 mg/kg Oral: 80 to 320 mg once a day
Sotalol (Betapace)	Oral: 240 to 480 mg/day, once a day I.V.: 10 to 20 mg
Timolol (Blocadren)	Oral: 15 to 45 mg (t.i.d. or q.i.d.) I.V.: 0.4 to 1 mg
Cardioselective beta blockers	
Acebutolol (Sectral)	Oral: 200 to 400 mg t.i.d.; maximum dose is 900 mg I.V.: 12.5 to 50 mg
Atenolol (Tenormin)	Oral: 100 mg once a day or 25 mg b.i.d. I.V.: 5 to 10 mg
Metoprolol (Betaloc, Lopressor)	Oral: 50 to 100 mg b.i.d. or t.i.d.; maximum dose is 200 mg I.V.: 5 to 15 mg
Vasodilatory beta blockers	
Celiprolol (Selecor)	Oral: 400 mg once a day
Labetalol (Trandate)	Oral: 300 to 600 mg/day, t.i.d.; maximum dose is 2,400 mg/day I.V.: 1 to 2 mg/kg for severe hypertension
Pindolol (Visken)	Oral: 2.5 to 7.5 mg t.i.d.

receptors in the heart. They have an intrinsic sympatholytic activity and lower the resting heart rate and the inotropic state of the myocardium. These drugs include acebutolol, atenolol, and metoprolol.
• Vasodilatory beta blockers obstruct beta-2 receptors in vascular smooth muscles, preventing vasospasm. These drugs include celiprolol, labetalol, and pindolol.

Dosage

Beta blockers may be administered orally or intravenously. (See *Dosages for class II antiarrhythmics*.)

Characteristic ECG changes

If your patient is receiving a beta blocker, you may note these changes on his ECG:
• prolonged PR interval
• shortened QT interval
• decreased heart rate.

Class II antiarrhythmics: Effects on the ECG

These drugs produce the following electrocardiogram (ECG) changes: a slightly prolonged PR interval and a slightly shortened QT interval.

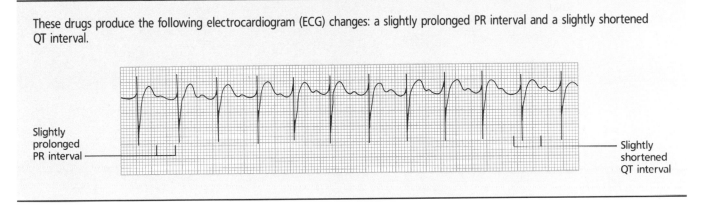

Slightly prolonged PR interval

Slightly shortened QT interval

Beta blockers can block the SA and AV nodes as well as the bundle branches. (See *Class II antiarrhythmics: Effects on the ECG.*)

Nursing considerations

• Avoid giving class II antiarrhythmics to patients with severe bradycardia, high-degree heart block, left ventricular failure, and certain peripheral vascular diseases.
• Use vasodilatory beta blockers cautiously in patients with asthma, hypertension, certain types of peripheral vascular disease, or conditions that cause a reactive pulmonary vascular bed.
• During therapy, monitor the patient for adverse effects, such as bronchospasm, fatigue, impotence, insomnia, nightmares and, in diabetic patients, hypoglycemia. Adverse cardiovascular reactions include decreased myocardial contractility, heart failure, sinus bradycardia, asystole, and AV block.
• After therapy, observe the patient for a rebound effect — an increased sensitivity to catecholamines following the withdrawal of beta blockers. In a patient with ischemic heart disease, an abrupt withdrawal can precipitate angina pectoris, MI, or arrhythmias.
• Caution the patient not to abruptly stop this drug without consulting his doctor because of the potential for a rebound effect.

Class III antiarrhythmics

Drugs in this class — amiodarone, bretylium, and sotalol — prolong repolarization and increase the duration of the action potential.

Class III drugs produce an antifibrillatory action by prolonging the refractory period, thus slowing the rate of ventricular tachycardia. Keep in mind that these drugs have differing pharmacologic actions and indications; therefore, they're not readily interchangeable.

Amiodarone

This drug treats patients with life-threatening ventricular arrhythmias that are unresponsive to other antiarrhythmics. Because of the risk of serious toxicity, amiodarone is contraindicated for treating PVCs.

Dosage
For rapid control of an arrhythmia, you'll typically administer 1,200 to 1,600 mg P.O. daily in two divided doses for 1 to 2 weeks. Then you'll give 400 to 800 mg daily for 1 to 3 weeks, followed by 200 to 400 mg once a day as a maintenance dose.

Class III antiarrhythmics: Effects on the ECG

These drugs produce the following electrocardiogram (ECG) changes: a prolonged PR interval, a widened or normal QRS complex, and a prolonged QT interval.

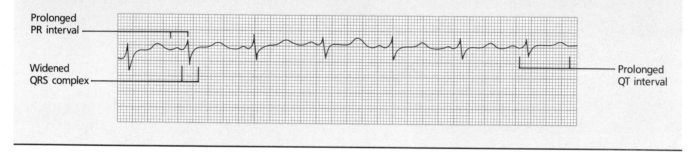

Prolonged PR interval

Widened QRS complex

Prolonged QT interval

Characteristic ECG changes

As with other class III agents, amiodarone causes the following:
• prolonged PR interval
• usually widened QRS complex
• prolonged QT interval.
You also may note T-wave changes and increased U-wave amplitude. (See *Class III antiarrhythmics: Effects on the ECG.*)

Amiodarone produces numerous electrophysiologic effects. It prolongs the action potential in cardiac tissues and bypass tracts. It also slightly reduces depolarization during phase 0 of the action potential, reflecting an inhibition of sodium channels. The drug depresses sinus node automaticity and prolongs conduction and refractoriness in the AV node. Plus, amiodarone blocks adrenergic receptors, causing vasodilation in coronary and peripheral vessels.

Nursing considerations

• Use amiodarone cautiously in patients who are taking digoxin or phenytoin concurrently because amiodarone can elevate blood levels of these drugs.
• Amiodarone can potentiate the effects of warfarin, so be alert for easy bruising or bleeding in patients receiving concurrent warfarin therapy.
• Pulmonary fibrosis is the most dangerous adverse effect of amiodarone, so periodically evaluate the patient's pulmonary status. This is especially important if he has preexisting pulmonary disease or is receiving long-term or high-dose amiodarone therapy.
• Instruct the patient to wear a sunscreen because the drug commonly causes photosensitivity.
• If the patient develops pseudocyanosis, which usually appears as a bluish discoloration of the facial skin, reassure him that this drug reaction isn't harmful.

Bretylium

The main indications for this drug are recurrent ventricular fibrillation and ventricular tachycardia that are refractory to lidocaine therapy and mechanical cardioversion.

Bretylium works by binding with the sympathetic neurons to cause chemical sympathectomy. That is, the drug initially releases stored norepinephrine from synaptic terminals, then inhibits further release.

Dosage

You'll administer bretylium I.V. The initial loading dose is 5 mg/kg. If the patient doesn't develop hypotension, you can increase the infusion rate to 10 mg/kg. After the loading dose, give a continuous drip of 1 to 2 mg/minute, as ordered.

Characteristic ECG changes

Like amiodarone, bretylium markedly prolongs repolarization. Typically, you'll observe a prolonged QT interval. Bretylium also lengthens the action potential in Purkinje fibers and exerts an inhibitory effect on nodal and conduction tissue.

Nursing considerations

• Because the initial dose of bretylium can trigger hypotension, administer the drug slowly. Check the patient's blood pressure; if hypotension doesn't develop, you may administer the drug faster.
• In some patients, you may notice an initial rise in blood pressure. Usually, this is a transient response that stems from a drug-induced release of norepinephrine from sympathetic nerve terminals.

Sotalol

This investigational drug is used to treat ventricular arrhythmias unresponsive to other antiarrhythmic drugs. It has both class II and III antiarrhythmic properties; in other words, it acts as both a beta blocker and an antiarrhythmic drug that prolongs repolarization.

Well tolerated for long-term therapy, sotalol is especially useful for hypertensive patients with arrhythmias, such as those with hypertrophic cardiomyopathy.

Dosage

Because sotalol is an investigational drug in the United States, its dosage requirements haven't been established. Given orally, typical dosages range from 200 to 600 mg daily.

Characteristic ECG changes

Typically, you'll observe a prolonged QT interval in patients receiving sotalol.

Nursing considerations

• If the patient is receiving diuretic therapy, monitor his potassium level closely. If hypokalemia develops, sotalol may trigger proarrhythmias.
• Because sotalol may induce torsades de

pointes, monitor the ECG for progressive lengthening of the QT interval and prominent U waves—two important warning signs of this proarrhythmia.
• Be aware that the effect of sotalol on the QT interval may be potentiated by other drugs that prolong repolarization, such as quinidine and amiodarone.

Class IV antiarrhythmics

Drugs in this class—verapamil, diltiazem, adenosine, and nifedipine—are calcium channel blockers. These drugs depress phase 4 depolarization and lengthen phases 1 and 2 of repolarization.

Class IV drugs predominantly affect the SA and AV nodal tissues. In these tissues, depolarization depends on slow calcium channels, rather than fast sodium channels. Calcium channel blockers produce a negative inotropic and vasodilatory effect.

Verapamil

This calcium antagonist is the drug of choice for paroxysmal SVT because of its ability to inhibit depolarization in the AV nodal tissue. Plus, in atrial fibrillation and flutter, verapamil reduces the ventricular response.

Dosage and pharmacodynamics

If oral verapamil is ordered, you'll give 80 to 120 mg three times daily. The dosage for slow-release preparations is 240 to 360 mg daily.

If I.V. verapamil is ordered, you'll give a bolus of 5 to 10 mg (0.1 to 0.15 mg/kg) over 1 minute. Repeat this dose after 10 minutes.

Characteristic ECG changes

When a patient is receiving verapamil, you may note the following ECG changes:
• prolonged PR interval

Class IV antiarrhythmics: Effects on the ECG

This class of antiarrhythmics lengthens the PR interval on the electrocardiogram (ECG).

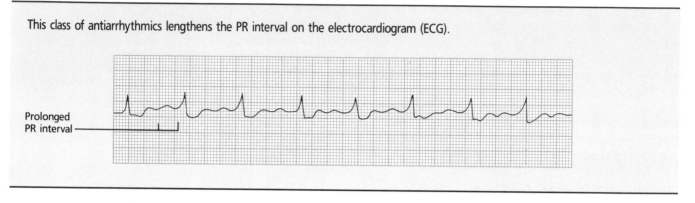

Prolonged PR interval

● decreased heart rate.
Be alert for severe bradycardia, especially in patients with depressed automaticity or AV nodal conduction disorders. (See *Class IV antiarrhythmics: Effects on the ECG.*)

Nursing considerations
● Use verapamil with caution in patients receiving beta blockers or disopyramide. This combination of drugs may cause arrhythmias.
● Also use verapamil cautiously in patients receiving concurrent digoxin therapy. Verapamil can elevate blood levels of digoxin, potentiating AV blockade.
● If the patient is receiving I.V. verapamil, monitor him for hypotension. Usually, this adverse reaction peaks within 5 minutes and resolves in 10 to 12 minutes.
● Patients who have a marked reduction in ventricular rate may experience PVCs. Monitor closely.
● The patient may experience constipation. Administer a stool softener, as needed.

Diltiazem

Although similar to verapamil, diltiazem has a greater effect on SA nodal tissue than on AV nodal tissue, so it's more likely than verapamil to decrease the heart rate. Diltiazem has a mild negative inotropic effect and a peripheral vasodilatory effect. Its antiarrhythmic action

stems from its ability to block calcium entry into the AV nodal tissue and to prolong the effective refractory period. It's used to treat paroxysmal SVT and may be given by continuous I.V. infusion to treat atrial fibrillation or flutter.

Dosage and pharmacodynamics
The usual dosage of diltiazem is 0.25 mg/kg I.V. bolus over 2 minutes. Most patients receive 20 mg. If no response is seen, give a second dose in 15 minutes or start a continuous I.V. infusion of 10 mg/hour.

Characteristic ECG changes
When a patient is receiving diltiazem, you may observe the following ECG changes:
● prolonged PR interval (because of reduced AV conduction)
● decreased heart rate (in patients with preexisting sinus node dysfunction, possibly severe bradycardia). The drug is contraindicated in patients with sick sinus syndrome and shouldn't be given to patients with second- or third-degree heart block unless a functioning pacemaker is present.

Nursing considerations
● Use the drug cautiously in patients receiving beta blockers or digitalis.
● The drug is compatible with the following I.V. solutions: dextrose 5% in water, 0.9% sodium chloride, and D_5W in 0.45% sodium chloride.
● Injection is compatible with furosemide.

Adenosine

The drug of choice for paroxysmal SVT, adenosine inhibits sinus and AV nodal conduction.

Dosage
Give adenosine in a rapid I.V. bolus of 6 mg. If the antiarrhythmic effect isn't achieved in 1 to 2 minutes, give a 12-mg bolus.

Characteristic ECG changes
If your patient is receiving adenosine, you may note the following ECG changes:
• decreased heart rate (in patients with preexisting sinus node dysfunction, possibly severe bradycardia)
• transient premature atrial or ventricular beats
• AV block.

Occasionally, you may observe ventricular pauses exceeding 2 seconds.

Nursing considerations
• Administering adenosine in a rapid I.V. bolus maximizes its effects on AV nodal tissue. You should see an immediate antiarrhythmic effect.
• Adenosine has a half-life of only 10 to 30 seconds, so adverse effects may be transient.

Nifedipine

This calcium antagonist has powerful arterial vasodilator effects. Its antiarrhythmic action reflects its ability to improve ischemic tissue by vasodilation of coronary arteries.

Dosage
The dosage for nifedipine depends on its indications.

Characteristic ECG changes
When a patient is receiving nifedipine, you may note the following ECG changes:
• prolonged PR interval
• decreased heart rate.

Nursing considerations
• Instruct the patient in the bite-and-swallow method of administration to ensure rapid absorption of the drug.
• Observe the patient for hypotension, which may develop as an adverse reaction within 20 minutes of oral ingestion and within 5 minutes of sublingual administration.

Treatment

Because nearly all antiarrhythmic drugs can trigger proarrhythmias, the doctor must weigh the risks of drug therapy before ordering an antiarrhythmic. Symptomatic or life-threatening arrhythmias require treatment, but asymptomatic PVCs or nonsustained ventricular tachycardia aren't always treated.

As a bedside nurse, you'll need to monitor the patient closely to detect proarrhythmias. If you see significant changes on a patient's ECG, notify the doctor immediately.

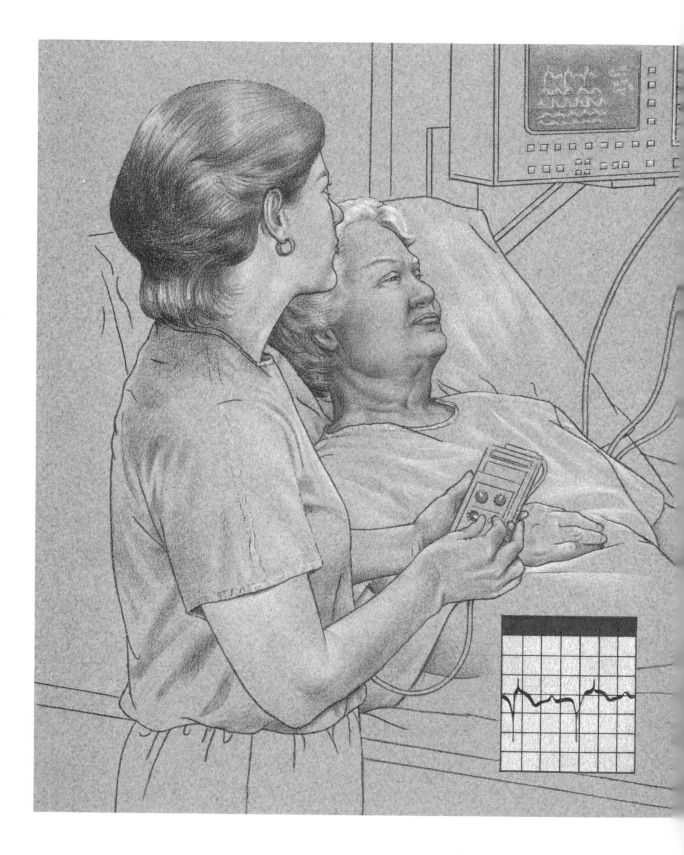

CHAPTER 13

Cardiac pacemakers

Cardiac pacing has undergone dramatic changes since 1952, when patients first received external pacemakers. Modern pacemakers are implantable, synchronized, rate-responsive, dual-chambered, and multiprogrammable. More than 200,000 are implanted every year in patients who have aberrant heart rhythms.

Of course, caring for a patient with a sophisticated pacemaker requires advanced nursing skills. And one of the most important is interpreting the patient's electrocardiogram (ECG) to evaluate pacemaker function. By correctly reading an ECG, you can detect pacemaker problems and intervene early.

This chapter will help you detect such problems and guide your interventions. It begins with a review of some fundamentals of pacemakers, including indications, general ECG characteristics, pacemaker components, and pacemaker placement. Next comes a section spelling out various pacemaker codes and modes. Then you'll find a section on the common types of pacemakers. The discussion here covers advantages and disadvantages as well as ECG characteristics. The chapter's last section explains how to use the ECG to evaluate pacemaker function.

Pacemaker basics

Essentially, a pacemaker electrically stimulates myocardial depolarization and prompts mechanical contraction when the heart fails to do so on its own. A doctor may recommend a pacemaker for such abnormalities as bradyarrhythmia, heart block, or symptomatic supraventricular tachycardia (SVT) that fails to respond to other therapy.

The doctor prescribes a certain type of pacemaker—permanent or temporary—based on the characteristics and permanence of the patient's arrhythmia as well as his symptoms, age, general health, and underlying heart disease.

A patient who needs a permanent pacemaker may have an arrhythmia associated with syncope, hypotension, dyspnea, angina, ectopy, or changes in level of consciousness. Common arrhythmias that warrant permanent pacemaker insertion include:
• symptomatic ventricular bradyarrhythmias that reduce cardiac output
• recurrent or permanent asymptomatic complete atrioventricular (AV) block with a ventricular rate under 40 beats/minute
• symptomatic second-degree AV block
• chronic bifascicular or trifascicular block
• sinus arrest or pauses exceeding 2½ seconds
• sick sinus syndrome
• atrial flutter or fibrillation with a ventricular response under 40 beats/minute
• bradyarrhythmias induced by drugs to control tachyarrhythmias.

To restore or maintain hemodynamic stability during a transient arrhythmia, a doctor may order a temporary pacemaker, especially if the arrhythmia results from a myocardial infarction (MI), drug toxicity, or thoracotomy. A temporary pacemaker is also indicated for a patient who has (or who's at high risk for) cardiac arrest; transient, symptomatic arrhythmias; hemodynamic instability from transient bradyarrhythmia; or transient tachyarrhythmia. Plus, a temporary pacemaker may be used for a patient at high risk for degenerative AV block. Temporary pacing may benefit a patient with asystole or SVT that doesn't respond to drugs. During SVT, the pacemaker interrupts or overrides the ectopic foci firing and halts the tachycardia, thereby restoring normal sinus rhythm.

Pacemaker-generated ECG characteristics

The pacemaker spike is the most striking change you'll see on the ECG of a patient with a pacemaker. The spike, which represents the electrical impulse the pacemaker sends to the heart, appears on the ECG tracing as a vertical line.
• If the electrode rests in or on the ventricle, the spike appears in front of every QRS complex stimulated by the pacemaker. The pacemaker causes ventricular activation similar to a left bundle-branch block. As a result, a wide QRS complex will follow a ventricular pacemaker spike.
• If the electrode lies in the atrium, a spike appears before every P wave stimulated by the pacemaker, showing that depolarization or capture (successful pacing) has occurred. The P wave may be inverted or differ in shape from the patient's intrinsic P wave.
• If electrodes are placed in both the atrium and ventricle, the spike appears before every P wave and QRS complex stimulated by the pacemaker.

Whenever you see a spike followed by a P wave or QRS complex, you know that capture has occurred in the chamber affected.

Pacemaker components

A pacemaker can be used temporarily or permanently. It can stimulate one or more heart chambers. Yet, whether it's ordered for a short period or a long time—and for whichever heart chamber—it will have these components: a pulse generator, a pacing lead (or leads), and an electrode tip (or tips).

Pulse generator

The pacemaker's power source is the pulse generator. This houses the battery and the circuitry that delivers an electrical charge to the heart. Containing lithium, the battery lasts about 10 years and, in a permanent pacemaker, must be replaced surgically. Longer-lasting (up to 40 years) nuclear batteries are being tested. The generator's circuitry is contained in a microchip. The brains of the pacemaker, this circuitry directs physiologic pacing.

Different types of pulse generators are available with different sensing and pacing capabilities. When the patient wears the pulse generator externally, the pacemaker is considered temporary; when the generator is implanted, the pacemaker is considered permanent.

Pacing leads and electrode tips

Once generated, an electrical impulse proceeds from the pulse generator, through the pacing lead (an insulated wire) and electrode tip, to the heart muscle. Single-chamber pacemakers have one pacing lead, usually in the right ventricle but sometimes in the right atrium or the left atrium or ventricle. Dual-chamber pacemakers have two pacing leads, one in the right atrium and one in the right ventricle. Sometimes, left-side chambers are used. Each pacing lead has one or two electrodes. A lead with one electrode is termed unipolar; a lead with two electrodes, bipolar. (See *Identifying pacing leads,* page 194.)

In general, a unipolar circuit is more sensitive to the heart's self-generated signals, whereas a bipolar circuit is less vulnerable to interference from external electrical fields and skeletal muscle stimulation. However, the bipolar lead is harder to implant. The electrode-tipped lead conducts endocardial impulses from the myocardium to the pacemaker's sensing circuitry and then conducts the electrical stimulus from the pulse generator to the myocardium.

Pacemaker placement

Whether the patient has a permanent or temporary pacemaker, the pacing lead follows a specific route—transmediastinal, transvenous, transthoracic, or transcutaneous.

Permanent pacing leads

In a permanent pacemaker, leads usually follow a transvenous route and are implanted endocardially. (See *Understanding endocardial lead placement,* page 195.) With the transvenous approach, patient morbidity remains low. With current lead designs, displacement rates also are low. Alternatively, leads can follow a transmediastinal or transthoracic route. These leads would be implanted epicardially.

A permanent pacemaker's pulse generator usually is implanted in a surgically created pocket in the subclavicular area. The generator also may be placed intra-abdominally, as with epicardial lead placement. In women, the generator may be placed beneath breast tissue.

Temporary pacing leads

The lead for a temporary pacemaker can be placed by the transmediastinal, transvenous, transthoracic, or transcutaneous routes. The lead can terminate on either the endocardial or epicardial surface. The pulse generator will be outside the patient's body. (For more information, see *Testing the stimulation threshold,* page 196.)

Transmediastinal placement

Epicardial leads attach to the outermost layer of the left or right ventricle by a transmediastinal route. Used less often than an endocardial lead, an epicardial lead may be appropriate for a patient with a dilated right ventricle (making endocardial lead adherence difficult) or for a patient who has had open-heart surgery.

To place this lead, the surgeon implants a sutureless corkscrew electrode on the epicardium of the left ventricle. Then he tunnels the lead subcutaneously to an external pulse generator. Epicardial leads also can be implanted permanently, in which case the generator is placed inside the abdomen. There, the genera-

Identifying pacing leads

A pacing lead may be unipolar (one electrode) or bipolar (two electrodes). The following illustrations show how a patient's electrocardiogram (ECG) tracing reflects which type of lead his pacemaker has.

Unipolar lead

In a unipolar pacing system, the electrode that rests in the myocardium (shown here in the right ventricle) acts as the negative pole, and the pulse generator acts as the positive pole. Because a relatively wide distance separates the two poles, you'll see tall spikes on the ECG (highlighted area).

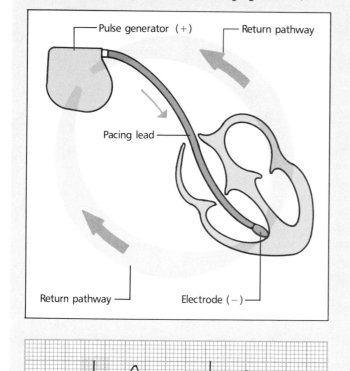

Bipolar lead

In a bipolar system, the two electrodes (shown here in the right ventricle) are just a few millimeters apart. Because the current travels only a short distance between positive and negative poles, you'll see a short spike on the ECG (highlighted area).

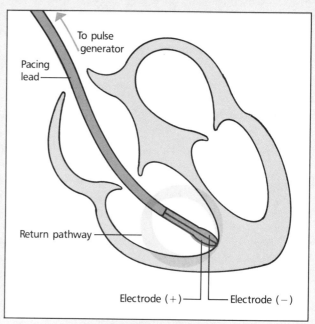

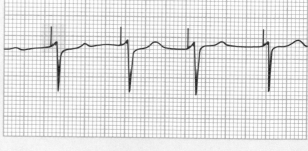

tor is less vulnerable to positional changes, such as bending. Transmediastinal placement of permanent epicardial leads requires the patient to undergo general anesthesia and another operation for lead repair or replacement.

A thoracotomy also may be performed to place the epicardial pacing lead. By this route, the surgeon can suture the electrode directly to the epicardium. Although the security of the lead attachment makes this approach advantageous, thoracotomy requires the patient to have a general anesthetic. For a permanent epicardial pacemaker, any repair or replacement of the lead requires repeated thoracotomy, thereby exposing the patient to complications related to pleural cavity entry.

Transvenous placement

Temporary transvenous leads can be placed percutaneously or by venous cutdown in the same way as permanent leads. The only difference is that the lead exits through the venous access site and connects to an external generator at the bedside. Many pulmonary artery catheters have an access port for right ventricular pacing leads. With this type of catheter, the doctor can thread the leadwire directly through the lumen into the right ventricle to initiate temporary pacing.

Transthoracic placement

In an emergency, the surgeon can insert a pacing lead percutaneously by an external transthoracic approach. The lead enters the right ventricle from a point inferior to the xiphoid process, or it enters the left ventricle apically via a pericardiocentesis-type needle. The external part of the pacing lead exiting through the chest wall attaches to an external generator. This approach is rarely used.

Transcutaneous placement

Also used in an emergency are large-surface skin electrodes, which can be placed on the anterior and posterior chest wall temporarily to stimulate cardiac pacing. Known as noninvasive transcutaneous cardiac pacing, this system has an external pulse generator and pacing cable which connects to the skin electrodes.

Understanding endocardial lead placement

Any patient receiving a permanent pacemaker will need surgery to insert the pacing lead or leads. The surgeon who implants the endocardial pacemaker usually selects a transvenous route (usually the subclavian, jugular, femoral, antecubital, or cephalic vein) and begins lead placement by inserting a catheter percutaneously or by venous cutdown.

Then, using a stylet and fluoroscopic guidance, he threads the catheter through the vein until the tip reaches the endocardium (the innermost layer of heart muscle).

For lead placement in the atrium, the catheter tip must lodge in the right atrium or the coronary sinus. For placement in the ventricle, the lead must lodge within the right ventricular apex in one of the interior muscular ridges (the trabeculae). See the illustration below.

Once the lead lies in the proper position, the surgeon secures the pulse generator in a subcutaneous pocket of tissue just below the right or left clavicle. Changing the generator's battery or microchip circuitry requires only a small shallow incision over the site and a quick component exchange.

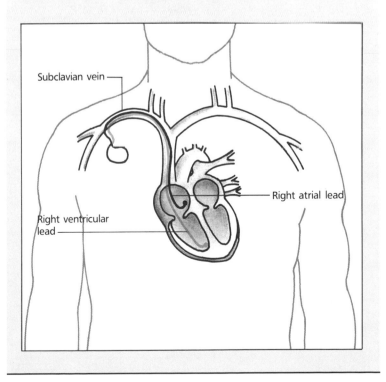

Testing the stimulation threshold

If your patient has a temporary pacemaker that's either actively operating or on standby, you'll need to check and document the stimulation threshold daily to ensure optimal functioning. The stimulation threshold is the minimum electrical stimulus needed to consistently evoke ventricular depolarization. Checking it involves assessing output and sensitivity.

Assessing output

Pacemaker output—measured in milliamperes (mA)—is the electrical energy (current) needed for ventricular depolarization. To assess function, begin by assessing capture:
• Increase the pacemaker rate to about 10 pulses/ minute faster than the patient's heart rate, and increase the mA to 10. The pacemaker should now be pacing on a 1:1 basis (electronically without intrinsic input) with each spike resulting in capture.
• Now, decrease mA until you lose capture; then increase mA just to the capture threshold—the point that restores capture. The ideal threshold is less than 1 mA.
• Next, set the mA dial for twice the threshold—usually about 3 mA—to ensure optimum capture without excessive energy output.
• Finally, restore the prescribed pacemaker rate.

Assessing sensitivity

Measured in millivolts (mV), sensitivity is the voltage needed to respond to the heart's electrical activity. To assess pacemaker sensitivity:
• Increase sensitivity to about 4 mV, making the pacemaker less sensitive. (A sensitivity of 20 mV would result in asynchronous pacing.)
• Decrease the pacemaker rate until it's about 10 pulses/minute less than the patient's own heart rate. You should see the patient's intrinsic rhythm traced on the electrocardiogram.
• Next, begin turning the sensitivity down until you reach the sensitivity threshold—the point at which the pacemaker no longer senses. (Sensitivity is set at roughly twice the threshold.)
• Finally, restore the pacemaker to its original heart rate.

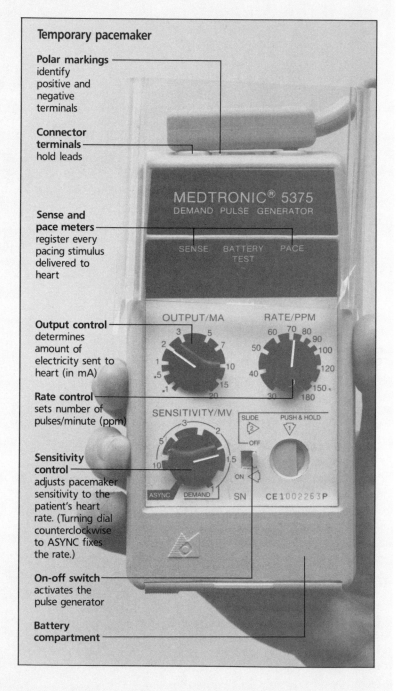

Temporary pacemaker

Polar markings identify positive and negative terminals

Connector terminals hold leads

MEDTRONIC® 5375
DEMAND PULSE GENERATOR

SENSE   BATTERY   PACE
TEST

Sense and pace meters register every pacing stimulus delivered to heart

OUTPUT/MA   RATE/PPM

Output control determines amount of electricity sent to heart (in mA)

Rate control sets number of pulses/minute (ppm)

SENSITIVITY/MV

Sensitivity control adjusts pacemaker sensitivity to the patient's heart rate. (Turning dial counterclockwise to ASYNC fixes the rate.)

On-off switch activates the pulse generator

Battery compartment

Besides its effectiveness when transvenous pacing is contraindicated—for example with coagulation problems, right ventricular MI, or sepsis—transcutaneous pacing has several advantages:
• It can be connected safely and quickly without a doctor.
• It supports the patient and controls arrhythmias until an appropriate pacemaker can be implanted.
• It serves prophylactically—for example, during patient transport, cardiac catheterization, elective cardioversion, and during insertion of a pulmonary artery catheter for a patient with an MI and bundle-branch block.

At times, however, transcutaneous pacing is impractical, especially if the patient has a large chest or extensive chest muscle mass, which requires the pacing impulse to travel too far for myocardial depolarization. Then, even if depolarization occurs, the increased energy required to generate capture causes the patient too much pain.

Transcutaneous pacing is also ineffective for patients with metabolic acidosis or myocardial ischemia because acidotic or ischemic tissue requires more electrical stimulus for depolarization than the pacing system can provide. Nor can this system be used during surgery involving electrocautery or electromagnetic or radio frequency interferences. An additional impracticality of this pacemaker in some patients is intense pain resulting from skeletal muscle stimulation and necessitating sedation or analgesia.

Pacemaker codes and modes

Once the lead or leads are placed and connected to the pulse generator, the pacemaker can begin its programmed functions. A synchronous (on demand) pacemaker program supports heart rate by responding to the heart's intrinsic electrical activity. An asynchronous (fixed-rate) pacemaker program stimulates the heart at a fixed, preset rate unrelated to intrinsic electrical activity.

A proliferation of pacemaker programs (more than 200 exist today) prompted several professional organizations to devise a coding system to describe the functional capabilities (or modes) of various pacemakers. Initially, a system was proposed by the Inter-Society Commission for Heart Disease Resources and revised by the North American Society of Pacing and Electrophysiology and the British Pacing and Electrophysiology group. The system is known by the letters NBG (derived from the contributing societies).

The NBG codes have five letters. The first three letters are associated exclusively with antibradyarrhythmia pacing. The letter "O" (none) is used in the first three letters to code antitachycardia devices because they don't have antibradyarrhythmia pacing capabilities.

First letter
The first letter identifies the heart chamber being paced. This letter may be:
• V for ventricle
• A for atrium
• D for dual (ventricle and atrium)
• O for none.

Second letter
The second letter indicates the heart chamber for which the pacemaker senses intrinsic activity.

The letter indicating the heart chamber being sensed may be:
• V for ventricle
• A for atrium
• D for dual (ventricle and atrium)
• O for none (a nonsensing pacemaker works asynchronously—or at a fixed rate).

Third letter
This letter indicates how the pulse generator responds to sensing the atrial activity (P wave) or ventricular activity (QRS complex). This letter may be:
• T for triggers pacing. In a VAT mode, for example, the chamber paced is the ventricle and the chamber sensed is the atrium. The pace-

maker triggers a ventricular impulse in synchrony with sensed atrial activity.

• I for inhibits pacing. If the pulse generator senses myocardial activity—depending on the chamber being sensed—the pacemaker won't fire but will reset. In VVI pacing, for instance, the pacemaker both paces and senses ventricular activity; when the pacemaker senses intrinsic ventricular activity, it inhibits extrinsic pacing and resets itself.

• D for dual triggering and inhibiting. In the DDD mode, the pulse generator is inhibited by any intrinsic atrial or ventricular activity, whereas in the VDD mode pacing, the pulse generator is inhibited only by intrinsic ventricular activity (because only ventricular pacing occurs). Additionally, in both the DDD and VDD modes, atrial-sensed activity triggers ventricular pacing.

• O for none. The generator doesn't change its mode of functioning in response to sensed activity. VOO is fixed-rate ventricular pacing.

Fourth letter

The fourth letter describes additional pacemaker capabilities: its degree of programmability and its rate responsiveness (rate modulation). This letter may be:

• P for simple programmable. This pacemaker has one or two programmable parameters.

• M for multiprogrammable. This pacemaker has three or more programmable parameters. (For more information, see *Reprogramming a pacemaker.*)

• C for communicating functions, such as telemetry (the noninvasive transmission of data from the implanted generator to an external receiver).

• R for rate responsiveness. To achieve a near-normal hemodynamic status, the pacemaker can adjust its rate to fit the patient's metabolic needs. In this mode, a sensor modulates the pacing rate in response to a physiologic cue, not to sinoatrial (SA) node activity, because the sinus node is diseased. Sensors may be mechanical, thermal, chemical, or electrical. Mechanical sensors respond to body motion, vibration, pressure, impedance, or color changes; thermal sensors detect changes in central venous blood temperature; chemical

sensors measure central venous pH; and electrical sensors measure changes in the heart's electrical activity.

Fifth letter

The fifth letter identifies how the pacemaker reacts to tachycardia. This letter may be:

• P for pacing. In antitachycardial pacing, the pulse generator introduces a stimulus prematurely to prevent the preceding beat from completing reentry and thereby halting the tachyarrhythmia. This can be done in several ways, one of which involves pacing the heart moderately faster (overdriving) than the intrinsic rate for a specific period. (*Caution*: Any type of induced rapid pacing can produce tachyarrhythmic acceleration or deterioration of the arrhythmia into ventricular fibrillation.)

• S for shock. An automatic implantable cardioverter-defibrillator (AICD) both identifies and terminates ventricular tachycardia. Once the sensing circuit analyzes the QRS complex activity and the heart rate, the AICD generates a shock. The AICD is implanted mainly in patients with refractory ventricular arrhythmias.

• D for dual (pacing and shock).

Common types of pacemakers

Pacemakers are commonly known by their programmed function and by the number of heart chambers (single-chamber or dual-chamber) having a pacing lead.

A single-chamber pacemaker has one pacing lead in one heart chamber—either the left or right atrium or ventricle. A dual-chamber pacemaker has two pacing leads—one in the right atrium and one in the right ventricle. Both pacemaker types have distinct features, advantages and disadvantages, and ECG characteristics.

Reprogramming a pacemaker

To meet a patient's changing needs, today's permanent pacemakers can be readjusted quickly and noninvasively.

Typical changes
Commonly programmable functions include rate, mode, pulse width, output, sensitivity, atrioventricular interval, upper rate limit, and lower rate limit. Refractory period (the interval in which the pacemaker's sensing mechanism becomes completely or partially nonresponsive to cardiac activity) and hysteresis (a prolonged pause interval intended to give the heart a chance to beat spontaneously) are usually programmable as well.

Keying in
To reprogram the pacemaker, an operator (a doctor or a nurse with advanced skills) places the programmer on the patient's thorax over the implanted pulse generator. She then initiates the desired changes by pressing the appropriate function keys. Once "keyed in," the coded information is transmitted to the pulse generator (by magnetic field or a selected radio frequency), where the changes are affixed in the circuitry.

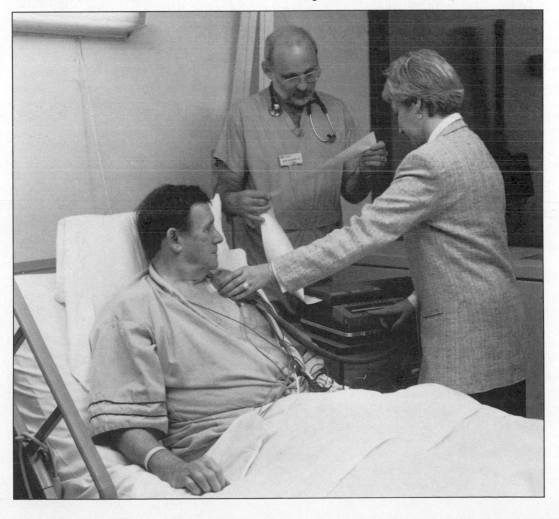

Single-chamber pacemakers

Typical single-chamber pacemakers include the ventricular demand (VVI) pacemaker and the atrial demand (AAI) pacemaker. (*Note:* The letters are the first three letters of the pacemaker's coded program.)

VVI pacemaker

The most common single-chamber pacemaker, the VVI has one lead in the right ventricle. As denoted by VVI, it both paces and senses ventricular activity (QRS complex). When it senses intrinsic ventricular activity, it can inhibit ventricular pacing and reset itself.

Advantages and disadvantages

This pacing mode may benefit a patient with complete heart block who doesn't need the hemodynamic benefit of atrial kick, who relies on the pacemaker stimulus infrequently, who is sedentary, or who would be at risk of runaway pacing from more sophisticated modes. Other risks include higher incidences of oversensing or undersensing.

The obvious limitation of this pacing is its lack of atrial kick, which can decrease cardiac output. Additionally, simultaneous atrial and ventricular contraction (from intrinsic atrial activity and paced ventricular activity) can cause mitral and tricuspid regurgitation and subsequent dyspnea.

ECG characteristics

If the patient's ventricular rate falls below the programmed pacemaker rate, the pacemaker delivers an impulse to the ventricle (to guard against bradycardia). Preceding the QRS complex, which indicates ventricular depolarization, you'll see a spike. And although you may see P waves on the ECG, this pacing mode won't sense or respond to them. (See *Where pacemaker spikes appear.*)

AAI pacemaker

Another single-chamber pacemaker, the AAI has one lead in the right atrium. Sometimes known as an atrial demand-inhibiting pacemaker, the AAI paces and senses the atrial chamber. What's more, it inhibits pacing upon sensing spontaneous atrial activity (P wave) and resets itself. In AAI pacing, the heart is responsible for conduction of the P wave past the AV node to the ventricles.

Advantages and disadvantages

AAI mode pacing may benefit a patient who has sick sinus syndrome but who doesn't have concomitant His-Purkinje disease, as long as his hemodynamic status is improved by atrial contribution to cardiac output. Sick sinus syndrome encompasses any abnormal discharge of the SA node that results in bradycardias, blocks, or escapes (such as SA arrest, SA exit block, or bradycardia-tachycardia syndrome). AAI pacing restores AV synchrony and improves cardiac output.

AAI pacing isn't effective, however, for a patient with atrial fibrillation because it doesn't prompt atrial depolarization. Nor is this pacing mode beneficial for a patient with AV block because the heart is responsible for conduction of the P wave through the AV node to the ventricles. Additionally, AAI pacing doesn't protect the patient against ventricular bradycardias.

ECG characteristics

If the patient's atrial rate falls below the pacemaker's programmed rate, the pacemaker delivers an impulse to the atrium (to guard against bradycardia). You'll see a pacemaker spike followed by a P wave or a captured P wave. The normal QRS complex that follows indicates that the heart's AV node conducted the impulse to the ventricle.

Dual-chamber pacemakers

These devices have two leads — one in the right atrium and one in the right ventricle. They include pacemakers programmed in the DVI, the VDD, and the DDD modes, as well as many others.

DVI pacemaker

Also known as an AV-sequential pacemaker, the DVI pacemaker paces the atrium and ventricle consecutively though it senses only ven-

Where pacemaker spikes appear

These electrocardiogram (ECG) waveforms show the relationship between the position of the spike caused by pacemaker activity and the heart chamber being paced in the pacing modes VVI, AAI, DVI, VDD, and DDD.

VVI pacemaker

With ventricular pacing, the spike appears before the QRS complex. This ECG shows the pacemaker in a ventricular pacing mode. There is no sensed intrinsic ventricular activity so the pacemaker fires in the ventricle to maintain the programmed heart rate.

AAI pacemaker

With atrial pacing, the spike appears before the P wave. This pacemaker senses and paces the atrium. The heart is responsible for conduction of the P wave past the atrioventricular (AV) node to the ventricles. In this strip, the pacemaker is responsible for atrial depolarization as indicated by a spike in front of every P wave. Each atrial depolarization is conducted through the AV node to the ventricles, as shown by the QRS complex following each P wave.

DVI pacemaker

With a DVI pacemaker, you may see atrial spikes before, during, or after intrinsically triggered P waves. In a committed pacemaker, intrinsic ventricular depolarizations that occur during the programmed AV interval of the second and sixth beats don't inhibit the ventricular pacing stimuli.

In a noncommitted pacemaker, intrinsic ventricular depolarizations within the AV interval of beats 2 and 5 do inhibit the ventricular pacing stimuli.

Committed

Noncommitted

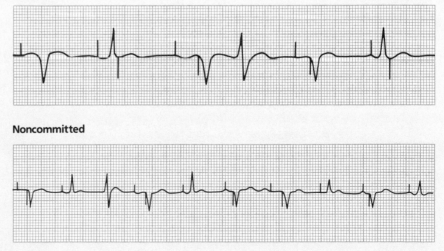

(continued)

Where pacemaker spikes appear *(continued)*

VDD pacemaker

With a VDD pacemaker, you'll see the patient's ventricular pacing rate change in association with intrinsic atrial activity, within the set pacemaker limits.

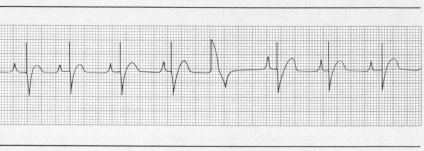

DDD pacemaker

With a DDD pacemaker, you may see a rhythm strip like this one, which shows automatic mode change (depending on the patient's intrinsic heart rhythm and rate. Complexes 1, 2, 4, 7, 11, 12, and 13 are in the atrial synchronous mode, with complexes 10 and 11 reflecting a maximum tracking rate of about 130 beats/minute. Complexes 3, 5, 8, and 10 (ventricular premature depolarizations) are sensed and inhibit the pacemaker. Complexes 6 and 9 are in the AV sequential mode that occurs at the escape rate of 70 beats/minute.

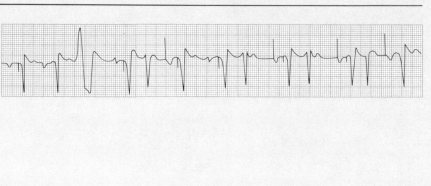

tricular activity. This means that both ventricular and atrial pacing depend on sensed ventricular activity. The DVI inhibits atrial and ventricular pacing after a sensed ventricular event.

Advantages and disadvantages

A patient who has sick sinus syndrome with His-Purkinje disease or a patient who has a high degree of AV block and who needs atrial kick would benefit from DVI pacing.

However, DVI pacing can't be used in the presence of atrial fibrillation because the atrial pacer would be unable to capture the atria due to fibrillatory intrinsic activity. Besides, this pacemaker performs no atrial sensing, so it's incapable of varying the atrial rate.

ECG characteristics

You'll notice atrial spikes before, during, or after intrinsic P waves because sensing occurs only in the ventricle. To inhibit the atrial stimulus, intrinsic ventricular activity must occur before the atrial spike is due.

The ECG can also identify the DVI pacemaker type—either committed or noncommitted (inhibited). Intrinsic ventricular activity generated within the AV interval (milliseconds between a sensed or paced atrial event and a paced ventricular event) causes a different ECG tracing with each type of pacemaker.

The committed pacemaker always transmits an impulse to the ventricle after atrial discharge and is inhibited only on the beat after the sensed ventricular activity. If ventricular activity is sensed, there will be no atrial or ventricular discharge. (A drawback to this system is that overuse of the pulse generator can limit its life.)

A noncommitted DVI pacemaker inhibits the ventricular pacing impulse if spontaneous ventricular activity occurs within the AV interval. A potential drawback of noncommitted pacing is self-inhibition.

VDD pacemaker
This pacemaker paces the ventricle and senses both atrial and ventricular activity. When it senses intrinsic atrial activity, it triggers ventricular pacing; when it senses intrinsic ventricular activity, it inhibits pacing and won't fire. This is also called P-synchronous pacing. The pacemaker's physiologic rate variability is made possible by tracking the SA node. The pacemaker senses atrial activity and fires the ventricular pacer in synchrony with atrial activity. This pacemaker inhibits pacing when the sensor notes intrinsic ventricular activity within the AV interval.

Advantages and disadvantages
This type of pacemaker may benefit a patient with third-degree heart block and a normal SA node whose hemodynamic status would benefit from atrial kick. VDD also may be selected for an active patient who needs physiologic rate variability.

This pacemaker is contraindicated for a patient with an SA node disease, such as atrial fibrillation or sick sinus syndrome.

ECG characteristics
Once the pacemaker senses atrial activity, it starts pacing the ventricle after a set time period that coincides with the AV interval. If it senses intrinsic ventricular activity, it inhibits pacing. Ventricular pacing occurs at a base rate if atrial activity is too slow or doesn't occur at all. Additionally, the ventricular pacing rate won't exceed a preset limit if intrinsic atrial activity is very fast.

You'll notice ventricular spikes after the preset AV delay. If an intrinsic QRS complex occurs during this time, the ventricular pacemaker will reset itself and you'll see no spike. The faster the intrinsic atrial rate the faster the

ventricular pacemaker will fire (to an upper rate limit), but only after the set AV interval.

DDD pacemaker
Fully automatic, the DDD pacemaker maintains AV synchrony at all times, mimics normal heart pacing most closely, and changes modes to fit the patient's needs. Of all pacemakers, the DDD has the most programmable parameters. It senses and synchronously paces the atrium and ventricle and varies the ventricular rate directly with the intrinsic atrial rate. It can pace a slow atrium or pace the ventricle if AV conduction is compromised. If the atrium depolarizes at a normal rate, but if AV conduction is compromised, the pacemaker can pace the ventricle in synchrony with the atrium. With spontaneous atrial or ventricular conduction, the pacemaker inhibits itself. Like the VDD, it has a programmed upper rate limit.

Advantages and disadvantages
A DDD pacemaker may help a patient who has severe AV block with or without sick sinus syndrome (but not a patient with atrial fibrillation).

The main drawback of this pacemaker is that its many capabilities make troubleshooting problems difficult.

ECG characteristics
A DDD pacemaker senses and synchronously paces the atria and ventricles, varying the ventricular rate according to the intrinsic atrial rate and the maximum rate limit. The ECG of a patient with a DDD pacemaker may show any of the following combinations:
• the patient's intrinsic rhythm without any pacemaker activity. This pattern results largely from the pacemaker's inhibitory function. Here's how. If the intrinsic atrial rate exceeds the pacer's lower rate, atrial pacing will be inhibited. If the intrinsic impulse can advance through the AV node to initiate ventricular depolarization before the programmed AV delay, the ventricular circuit will be inhibited. The ECG will show only the heart's intrinsic activity.
• an intrinsic P wave followed by a spike and a wide QRS complex (indicating ventricular depolarization). The tracing reflects atrial tracking.

LEAD OF CHOICE

Monitoring patients with pacemakers

When monitoring patients with pacemakers, use lead V_1 (MCL$_1$). The QRS morphology of the paced beat in this lead should be negative as in left bundle-branch block.

If the shape of the QRS complex of the paced beat becomes positive, the pacemaker leadwire in the right ventricle may have migrated to the outflow tract of the right ventricle or may have perforated the septum to lodge in the left ventricle.

Lead V$_1$

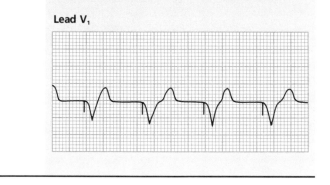

This occurs when the patient's intrinsic atrial rate exceeds the programmed lower rate limit but the impulse can't prompt ventricular depolarization. Then, ventricular pacing is triggered in response to the intrinsic atrial activity. The ventricular rate won't exceed the programmed upper rate limit.
• an intrinsic atrial rate that drops below the programmed atrial rate (indicating that the pulse generator initiated atrial pacing). If the atrial impulse can advance through the AV node to initiate ventricular depolarization before the programmed AV delay, then the ventricular circuit is inhibited. The ECG will show atrial pacing spikes followed by captured P waves, a normal PR interval, and an intrinsic QRS complex.
• no intrinsic activity in either the atria or ventricles (indicating that both are paced at the lower rate limit). The ECG will show atrial spikes and captured P waves, the programmed AV interval, and ventricular spikes and capture.

Evaluating pacemaker function

By assessing your patient's condition, you can detect how well he's adjusting to his pacemaker. And by evaluating his ECG, you can determine whether his pacemaker is working properly. (See *Monitoring patients with pacemakers*, and *Recognizing common pacemaker problems*.)

The most common undesirable effect of temporary or permanent pacemakers is extracardiac stimulation of the pectoral muscle. This results in twitching or stimulation of the diaphragm and causes hiccups. Decreasing the pulse width (the duration of the pacing pulse expressed in milliseconds) or voltage may eliminate this benign but bothersome side effect.

Interpreting the ECG

To evaluate how well your patient's pacemaker is working, start by asking yourself these questions:
• What is the current pacing mode?
• Is the system unipolar or bipolar?
• What are the programmed measurements?
• Is the patient having symptoms of decreased cardiac output?

Four-step method
Then use this four-step method to evaluate the atrial event, the AV interval, the ventricular event, and the ventriculoatrial (VA) interval.

Atrial event
Look at the morphology of the P wave. Now ask yourself these questions: Does this P wave reflect intrinsic atrial activity? Was it sensed? Is sensing a function of the programmed mode? What is the P wave's relationship to the QRS complex? Does it result from pacing? Does it show capture? What is the atrial pacing rate?

AV interval
Use this step only in dual-chamber pacing to evaluate the AV interval. Look at the ECG strip, and ask yourself these questions: Is this interval

Recognizing common pacemaker problems

You can detect some common pacemaker problems by using the electrocardiogram (ECG).

Failure to capture

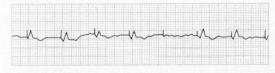

On this strip, the fifth ventricular spike isn't followed by a paced QRS complex.

SIGNS AND SYMPTOMS	POSSIBLE CAUSES	CORRECTIVE MEASURES
• ECG pacemaker spikes not followed by appropriate atrial or ventricular depolarization. If the pacemaker uses an atrial electrode, the spike won't be followed by a P wave; if the pacemaker uses a ventricular electrode, the spike won't be followed by a QRS complex. • Hypotension, light-headedness, fatigue, or extreme bradycardia from prolonged pause in cardiac activity • No response to magnet application, which should convert a synchronous pacemaker to an asynchronous one	• Lead dislodgment • Low pacemaker voltage • Dead battery • Fractured leadwire • Edema or scar tissue at electrode tip • Myocardial perforation with lead migration to an extracardiac position • Myocardial infarction at the leadwire	• Reposition or replace lead. • Reposition electrode tip. • Increase voltage. • Replace battery.

Failure to pace

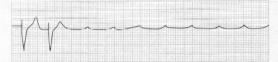

Here, the first two ventricular complexes are caused by the ventricular pacemaker. After the two complexes, there is no evidence of any ventricular pacing activity. As a result, this patient is asystolic.

SIGNS AND SYMPTOMS	POSSIBLE CAUSES	CORRECTIVE MEASURES
• No apparent pacemaker activity on the ECG • Hypotension, light-headedness, syncope, and bradycardia from prolonged ventricular standstill	• Incorrect connection of lead to generator (loose screws) • Broken or displaced leadwires • Pulse generator failure • Battery or circuit failure • "Crosstalk" between atrial and ventricular portions of dual-chamber pacemakers, which causes the atrial stimulus to be sensed by the ventricular sensor, thereby inhibiting the ventricular stimulus	• Repair connection or tighten terminal (if the patient has a temporary pacemaker). • Replace battery, generator, or lead.

(continued)

Recognizing common pacemaker problems *(continued)*

Failure to sense

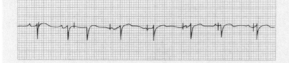

This ECG of a patient with an AAI pacemaker shows the pacemaker failing to sense intrinsic atrial activity. Atrial spikes in the second complex fall in the ST segment; the atrial spike in the seventh complex falls in the PR interval. P waves immediately following atrial spikes, which indicate capture, are associated with complexes IV, V, and VI. This indicates appropriate pacemaker activity.

SIGNS AND SYMPTOMS	POSSIBLE CAUSES	CORRECTIVE MEASURES
• ECG pacemaker spikes out of place; for example, in the ST segment, in the PR interval, or on the T wave • Palpitations or skipped beats • Ventricular tachycardia	• Lead dislodgment (most common) • Inappropriate lead placement • Increased sensing threshold caused by edema or fibrosis at electrode tip • Infarct • Drugs • Electrolyte disturbances • Fractured leadwire • Connector defect • Defective or dead battery	• Reposition lead, or position patient on his left side. • Replace battery and lead. • Tighten all connections. • Increase sensitivity setting.

Oversensing

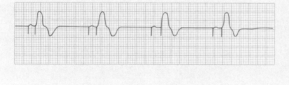

This ECG belongs to a patient with a DDD pacemaker. The lower rate limit is set for 60 beats/minute, and the pacemaker is firing at 43 beats/minute. The ventricular circuit is incorrectly sensing the large inverted T wave as ventricular activity, therefore inhibiting the pacemaker and resulting in the lower firing rate.

SIGNS AND SYMPTOMS	POSSIBLE CAUSES	CORRECTIVE MEASURES
• No paced beats on ECG even though the pacemaker's set rate exceeds the patient's spontaneous rate • Pacing at slower-than-set rate	• In unipolar pacemakers—sensing of skeletal muscle potentials generated by contraction of major pectoral muscles, causing inappropriate inhibition or firing • Electromagnetic interference (from power lines, radio or television transmitters, or other phenomena) • Sensing T waves or atrial activity • Pacemaker sensitivity set too high (most common)	• Lower sensitivity of a temporary pacemaker. • Reprogram a permanent pacemaker. • Place pacemaker in asynchronous mode (by applying a magnet or turning off sensitivity). • Insert bipolar lead.

Recognizing common pacemaker problems *(continued)*

Pacing at an altered rate

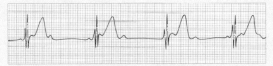

This ECG strip of a patient with a DDD pacemaker shows pacemaker-mediated tachycardia. Atrial tracking, reflected by the retrograde P wave, triggers ventricular activity at a tachycardic rate.

SIGNS AND SYMPTOMS	POSSIBLE CAUSES	CORRECTIVE MEASURES
• Tachycardia with pacemaker spike preceding each QRS complex (see highlighted area)	• Retrograde conduction through AV node (from dual-chamber pacing), which repolarizes atria and triggers rapid heart rates (most common)	• Reprogram pacemaker to atrial nonsensing mode. • Decrease heart rate by holding a magnet over pulse generator. This will convert pacer from synchronous to asynchronous mode until it can be reprogrammed (suitable only in an emergency).

Diaphragmatic pacing

This ECG strip shows a unipolar electrogram from the right ventricular pacing electrode, suggesting perforation of the myocardium. Note the positive R wave. The R to S ratio of the QRS complex is around 1.

SIGNS AND SYMPTOMS	POSSIBLE CAUSES	CORRECTIVE MEASURES
• Patient hiccups when pacemaker functions at set rate.	• Perforation of myocardium by leadwire • Output setting too high (in temporary pacemaker)	• Assess for myocardial perforation with a 12-lead ECG. (Endocardial lead should show left bundle-branch block with left axis deviation; epicardial lead, right bundle-branch block with a varying axis. Deviations suggest perforation.) • Decrease output setting (in temporary pacemaker) until hiccups subside.

a programmed value? If not, is the AV interval intrinsically inhibited?

Ventricular event

Look at the QRS complex on the ECG strip. Does its morphology reflect intrinsic ventricular activity? Was it sensed? Or does it result from pacing? Is sensing a function of the programmed mode? Does it show capture? What is the ventricular pacing rate?

VA interval

Use this step only to evaluate dual-chamber pacing. In this kind of pacemaker, the VA interval is the number of milliseconds between a sensed or paced ventricular event and a paced atrial event that immediately follows the QRS complex. Study the ECG strip and ask yourself: Does this tracing reflect a programmed value? If not, does the strip suggest an intrinsically inhibited atrial pacer?

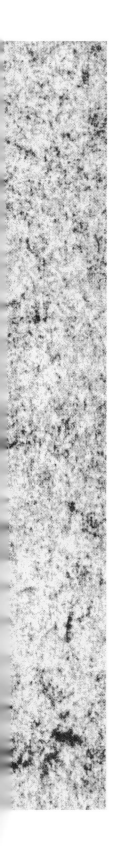

▶ **Suggested readings**

▶ **Advanced skilltest**

▶ **Index**

Suggested readings

Abedin, Z., and Conner, R. *12-Lead ECG Interpretation: The Self-Assessment Approach.* Philadelphia: W.B. Saunders Co., 1989.

Azuma, K., et al. "Hypokalemia Decreases Na⁺-K⁺-ATPase Alpha 2 but Not Alpha 1 Isoform Abundance in Heart, Muscle, and Brain," *American Journal of Physiology* 260(5 Pt 1):958-64, May 1991.

Boisaubin, E.V., et al. "Hypercalcemia of Advanced Malignancy: Decision Making and the Quality of Death," *The American Journal of Medical Sciences* 301(5):314-18, May 1991.

Braunwald, E. *Heart Disease: A Textbook of Cardiovascular Medicine,* 4th ed. Philadelphia: W.B. Saunders Co., 1992.

Cairns, C., et al. "Ionized Hypocalcemia during Prolonged Cardiac Arrest and Closed-Chest CPR in a Canine Model," *Annals of Emergency Medicine* 20(11):1178-82, November 1991.

Chou, T. *Electrocardiography in Clinical Practice,* 3rd ed. Philadelphia: W.B. Saunders Co., 1991.

Chung, E.K. *Electrocardiography: Self-Assessment.* East Norwalk, Conn.: Appleton & Lange, 1988.

Conover, M. *Understanding Electrocardiography, Arrhythmias and the 12-lead ECG,* 6th ed. St. Louis: Mosby-Year Book, Inc., 1992.

ECG Interpretation. Clinical Skillbuilders Series. Springhouse, Pa.: Springhouse Corp., 1990.

Friday, B.A., and Reinhart, R.A. "Magnesium Metabolism: A Case Report and Literature Review," *Critical Care Nurse* 11(5):62-72, May 1991.

Goldberger, A., and Goldberger, E. *Clinical Electrocardiography.* St Louis: C.V. Mosby Co., 1990.

Goldschlager, N., and Goldman, M. *Principles of Electrocardiography,* 13th ed. East Norwalk, Conn.: Appleton & Lange, 1989.

Gomes, J.A., and El-Sherif, N. "Atrioventricular Block: Mechanism, Clinical Presentation and Therapy," *Medical Clinics of North America* 68(4):955-67, July 1984.

Holtzman, G. "Magnesium," *Critical Care Nurse* 10(7):81-83, July-August 1990.

Hurst, J.W., et al. *The Heart,* 7th ed. New York: McGraw-Hill Book Co., 1990.

Huszar, R.J. *Basic Dysrhythmias: Interpretation and Management.* St. Louis: C.V. Mosby Co., 1988.

Innerarity, S. "Hyperkalemia Emergencies," *Critical Care Nursing Quarterly* 14(4):32-39, February 1992.

Karb, V. "Electrolyte Abnormalities and Drugs Which Commonly Cause Them," *Journal of Neuroscience Nursing* 21(2):125-29, April 1989.

Kay, G.N., and Bubien, R.S. *Clinical Management of Cardiac Arrhythmias.* Rockville, Md.: Aspen Pubs., Inc., 1991.

Kurtzman, N., et al."A Patient with Hyperkalemia and Metabolic Acidosis," *American Journal of Kidney Diseases* 15(4):333-56, April 1990.

Lagergren, H. "25 Years of Implanted Intracardiac Pacers," *Lancet* 1(8586):636-38, March 1988.

Mallette, L.E., et al. "Malignancy Hypercalcemia: Evaluation of Parathyroid Function and Response to Treatment," *American Journal of the Medical Sciences* 302(4):205-10, October 1991.

Martin, B., et al. "Hypomagnesemia in Elderly Hospital Admissions: A Study of Clinical Significance," *Quarterly Journal of Medicine* 78(286):177-84, February 1991.

McDermott, K.C., et al. "The Diagnosis and Management of Hypomagnesemia: A Unique Treatment Approach and Case Report," *Oncology Nursing Forum* 18(7):1145-51, September-October 1991.

Nattel, S., et al. "Actions of Intravenous Magnesium on Ventricular Arrhythmias Caused by Acute Myocardial Infarction," *Journal of Pharmacology and Experimental Therapeutics* 259(2):939-46, November 1991.

Rigolin, V., and Chap, L. "Extreme Hyperkalemia Induced by Drugs," *Postgraduate Medicine* 90(5):129-31, October 1991.

Salem, M., et al. "Hypomagnesemia Is a Frequent Finding in the Department in Patients with Chest Pain," *Archives of Internal Medicine* 151(1):2185-90, November 1991.

Schamroth, L. *An Introduction to Electrocardiography,* 7th ed. Boston: Blackwell Scientific Publications, 1990.

Sweetwood, H. *Clinical Electrocardiography for Nurses,* 2nd ed. Rockville, Md.: Aspen Pubs., Inc., 1988.

Vinsant, M.O., and Spence, M.I. *A Commonsense Approach to Coronary Care,* 5th ed. St. Louis: C.V. Mosby Co., 1989.

Wellens, H., and Conover, M. *The ECG in Emergency Decision Making.* Philadelphia: W.B. Saunders Co., 1992.

Wingate, S. *Cardiac Nursing: A Clinical Management and Patient Care Resource.* Rockville, Md.: Aspen Pubs., Inc., 1991.

Wrenn, K.D., et al. "The Ability of Physicians to Predict Hyperkalemia from the ECG," *Annals of Emergency Medicine* 20(11):1229-32, November 1991.

Advanced skilltest

This self-test presents case histories with related multiple-choice questions as well as general multiple-choice questions on interpreting electrocardiograms (ECGs). The questions begin on this page and continue to page 221. You'll find the answers and rationales on pages 222 and 223.

Case history questions

Mr. Vincent, age 74, is admitted to your unit after experiencing two episodes of syncope while at work. His blood pressure is 120/70 mm Hg, and his heart rate is 96 beats/minute. He has a history of coronary artery disease and hypertension that's controlled by diltiazem. You look at his rhythm strip, shown at right.

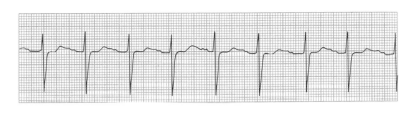

1. Mr. Vincent's initial rhythm strip indicates:

    a. sinus tachycardia.

    b. first-degree atrioventricular (AV) block.

    c. second-degree Type I AV block.

    d. third-degree AV block.

2. Using the small-block method for calculating heart rate, you'd find Mr. Vincent's ventricular rate to be:

    a. 80 beats/minute.

    b. 88 beats/minute.

    c. 94 beats/minute.

    d. 100 beats/minute.

3. On Mr. Vincent's rhythm strip, the QRS complex and the QT interval measure:

    a. 0.08 second and 0.30 second.

    b. 0.20 second and 0.42 second.

    c. 0.12 second and 0.28 second.

    d. 0.10 second and 0.42 second.

Two hours after Mr. Vincent is admitted, you observe the rhythm strip shown at right.

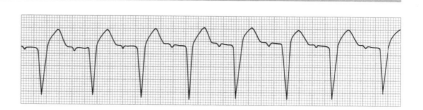

4. This rhythm strip indicates:

    a. left bundle-branch block.

    b. right bundle-branch block.

    c. left anterior hemiblock.

    d. left posterior hemiblock.

Within 3 hours, you notice that the QRS complexes have changed direction, as shown at right.

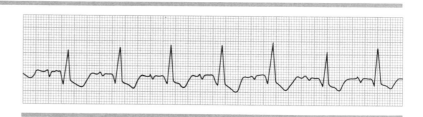

5. You'd interpret this change as an indication of:

    a. left bundle-branch block.

    b. right bundle-branch block.

    c. left anterior hemiblock.

    d. left posterior hemiblock.

6. The PR interval, QRS complex, and QT interval measure:

    a. 0.24 second, 0.20 second, and 0.38 second.

    b. 0.28 second, 0.16 second, and 0.40 second.

    c. 0.32 second, 0.18 second, and 0.52 second.

    d. 0.28 second, 0.16 second, and 0.44 second.

Mr. Vincent has a DDD permanent pace-maker inserted, and the implant work-sheet provides this information: low rate, 70 ppm; AV delay, 175 ms; upper rate limit, 110 ppm. Following insertion, you obtain this rhythm strip.

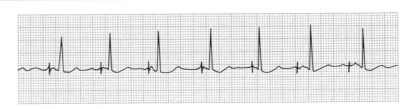

7. In which mode is the pacemaker functioning?
- a. AV sequential mode
- b. AAI mode
- c. VVI mode
- d. DOO mode

Three hours after the pacemaker is in-serted, you obtain this rhythm strip.

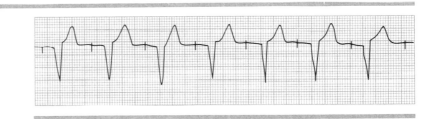

8. What's the current pacemaker mode?
- a. AV sequential mode
- b. AAI mode
- c. VVI mode
- d. Atrial tracking mode

9. The QRS complex measures:
- a. 0.08 second.
- b. 0.10 second.
- c. 0.12 second.
- d. 0.20 second.

10. The lead of choice for monitoring a patient with a pacemaker is:
- a. lead II.
- b. lead III.
- c. Lewis lead.
- d. lead MCL$_1$.

Mrs. Rogers, age 45, is admitted to your unit with palpitations and syncope. Her systolic blood pressure is 70 mm Hg, and her heart rate is 230 beats/minute. On admission, the following 12-lead ECG is obtained.

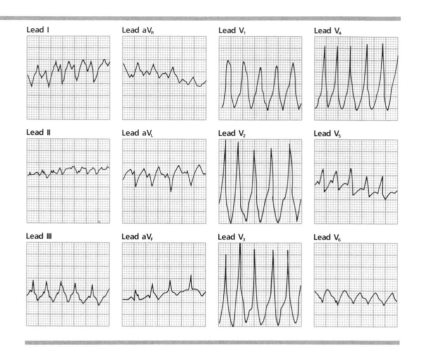

11. Based on Mrs. Rogers's signs and symptoms and your ECG findings, you'd expect the initial treatment to include:

    a. insertion of an overdrive pacemaker.

    b. cardioversion.

    c. administration of lidocaine.

    d. administration of verapamil.

12. Using the quadrant method, you'd determine the axis for this 12-lead ECG to be:

    a. extreme.

    b. left.

    c. normal.

    d. right.

13. Using the degree method, you'd determine the axis to be:

    a. − 30 degrees.

    b. + 150 degrees.

    c. + 60 degrees.

    d. − 60 degrees.

Mrs. Rogers responds to therapy, and another 12-lead ECG is obtained.

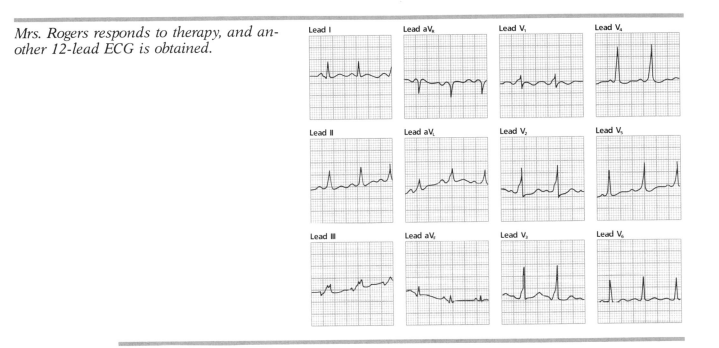

14. Using the quadrant method, you'd determine the axis to be:

    a. extreme.

    b. left.

    c. normal.

    d. right.

15. Using the degree method, you'd determine the axis to be:

    a. + 60 degrees.

    b. + 30 degrees.

    c. − 120 degrees.

    d. − 50 degrees.

16. Mrs. Rogers's underlying heart rhythm is:

    a. normal sinus rhythm.

    b. sinus tachycardia.

    c. first-degree AV block.

    d. atrial tachycardia.

17. In lead II, the PR interval measures:

    a. 0.10 second.

    b. 0.12 second.

    c. 0.20 second.

    d. 0.24 second.

18. In lead II, the QRS complex measures:

    a. 0.08 second.

    b. 0.10 second.

    c. 0.12 second.

    d. 0.14 second.

19. In lead II, the QT interval measures:

    a. 0.30 second.

    b. 0.32 second.

    c. 0.36 second.

    d. 0.50 second.

20. The upward sloping QRS complex, called a delta wave, indicates:

    a. hypothermia.

    b. hyperthermia.

    c. Wolff-Parkinson-White syndrome.

    d. AV block.

Mr. Nielson, age 60, is admitted to the cardiac care unit after developing chest pain while mowing his lawn. He has a history of myocardial infarction. His initial ECG, obtained in the emergency department, revealed ST elevation in the inferior and lateral wall leads. Now, 10 minutes later, the following 12-lead ECG is obtained.

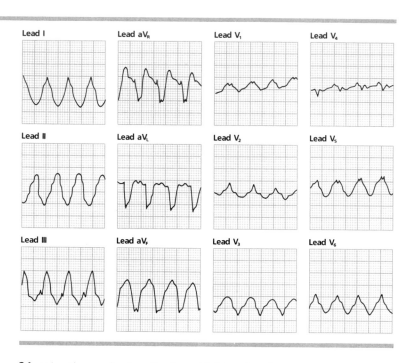

21. Using the quadrant method, you'd determine the axis to be:

         a. extreme.

         b. left.

         c. normal.

         d. right.

22. This 12-lead ECG indicates:

         a. supraventricular tachycardia.

         b. ventricular tachycardia.

23. In lead III, the QRS complex duration and the ventricular rate are:

         a. 0.10 second and 100 beats/minute.

         b. 0.16 second and 120 beats/minute.

         c. 0.20 second and 150 beats/minute.

         d. 0.24 second and 180 beats/minute.

Mrs. Jacobs, age 57, is admitted to your unit with palpitations and weakness. She tells you that her job is stressful, and she reports episodes of "fluttering" feelings in her chest. You look at her 12-lead ECG, which is shown at right.

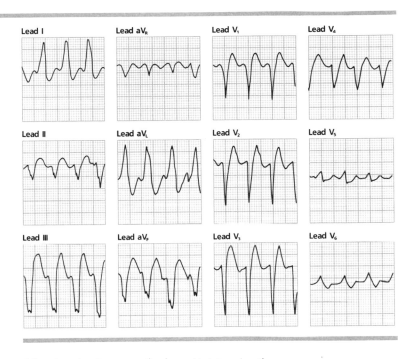

24. Using the degree method, you'd determine the axis to be:

        a.   − 60 degrees.

        b   + 150 degrees.

        c.   + 120 degrees.

        d.   − 30 degrees.

25. This 12-lead ECG indicates:

        a. supraventricular tachycardia.

        b. ventricular tachycardia.

After receiving 6 mg of adenosine by rapid I.V. push, Mrs. Jacobs's ECG changes from supraventricular tachycardia with a rate of 140 beats/minute to the ECG shown at right.

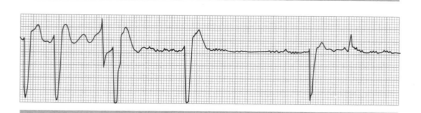

26. Which statement regarding the effects of adenosine is correct?

    a. Adenosine should have slowed the ventricular rate gradually, over a number of minutes.

    b. Because adenosine has an extremely short half-life, this is the anticipated effect.

    c. Because adenosine prolongs the QT interval, it shouldn't have produced periods of asystole.

    d. Adenosine interrupts the firing of the sinoatrial node but doesn't affect the AV node. Thus, the AV node should have fired as the pacemaker.

Mrs. Morse, age 50, is admitted to your unit with shortness of breath and tightness in her chest. Her health history includes hypothyroidism and diabetes mellitus. Her initial 12-lead ECG appears at right.

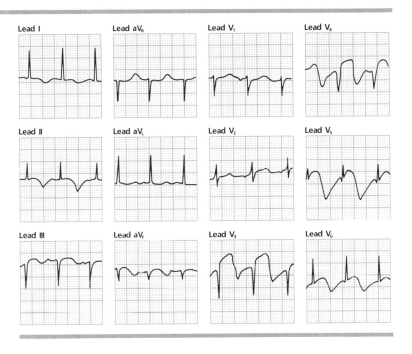

27. Infarction has occurred in which walls of the left ventricle?

    a. Anterior, inferior, and lateral walls

    b. Anterior, inferior, and posterior walls

    c. Inferior, lateral, and posterior walls

    d. Anterior, inferior, lateral, and posterior walls

28. Using the quadrant method, you'd determine the axis to be:

    a. extreme.

    b. left.

    c. normal.

    d. right.

29. Which leads in the adjacent 12-lead ECG show pathologic Q waves?

    a. Leads V_1, V_2, V_3, and V_4

    b. Leads I, aV_L, V_5, and V_6

    c. Leads II, III, and aV_F

    d. Leads aV_R, V_5, and V_6

30. These Q waves indicate old damage to which wall of the left ventricle?

    a. Anterior wall

    b. Inferior wall

    c. Lateral wall

    d. Posterior wall

31. Which coronary artery supplies the damaged ventricular wall?

    a. Circumflex artery

    b. Left anterior descending (LAD) artery

    c. Left main artery

    d. Right coronary artery

32. Which AV block is characterized by intermittent blocked beats, varying PR intervals, normal QRS complexes, and irregular R-R intervals?

    a. First-degree AV block

    b. Type I second-degree AV block

    c. Type II second-degree AV block

    d. Third-degree AV block

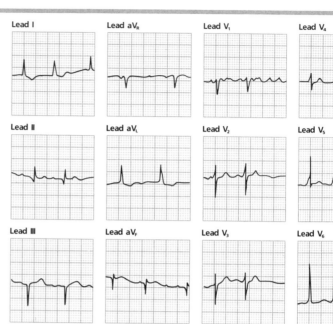

33. Which type of block does the adjacent 12-lead ECG show?

  a. Left bundle-branch block

  b. Right bundle-branch block

  c. Left anterior hemiblock

  d. Left posterior hemiblock

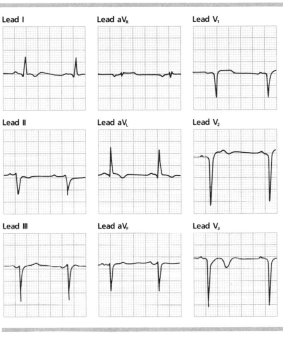

34. In the 12-lead ECG at right, obtained from a patient with episodic chest pain, the deep symmetrical T-wave inversion in leads V_2 through V_6 indicates:

  a. acute anterior wall infarction.

  b. preexcitation syndrome.

  c. Prinzmetal's angina.

  d. Wellens' syndrome.

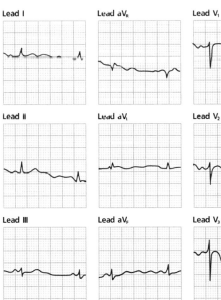

Answers and rationales

1. b. The atrial and ventricular rates are 90 beats/minute. The PR interval is 0.28 second and constant; the QRS complex duration is 0.10 second. A P wave precedes each QRS complex, and the rhythm is regular. The P wave is M-shaped.

2. b. The interval between two R waves is 17 small blocks. 1,500 ÷ 17 = 88 beats/minute.

3. d.

4. a. The QRS complex has a negative deflection and a duration of 0.14 second. This indicates that the energy of depolarization is traveling away from the positive pole of MCL_1, which sits on the right side of the heart. The blocked area is the last to depolarize, indicating that the left bundle is blocked.

5. b. The QRS complex duration is 0.16 second. The terminal part of the QRS complex in lead MCL_1 is positive. This indicates that the energy of depolarization is traveling toward the positive pole of MCL_1, which sits on the right side. The blocked area depolarizes last. Therefore, the right bundle is blocked.

6. d.

7. b. The atrial spike indicates that this pacemaker is firing in the atrium. The atrial capture and the impulse are conducted via the AV node to the ventricles, as indicated by the narrow QRS complex.

8. a. The atrial and ventricular spikes indicate that the pacemaker is functioning in the AV sequential mode. The ventricular spike is difficult to see on this ECG strip, but an important clue is the widened QRS complex. (Note that the QRS complex here is wider than the intrinsic QRS complex on the previous strip.) This may indicate that the filter on the monitor is filtering out the spike.

9. c. The QRS complex measures 3 small blocks. 3 × 0.04 = 0.12 second.

10. d. Lead MCL_1 allows you to verify captured beats that have a left bundle-branch block configuration. If the appearance of the QRS complex changes to a right bundle-branch block configuration, you would suspect lead migration.

11. b. This patient is experiencing hemodynamic instability; therefore, she requires cardioversion—the most efficient and appropriate therapy for terminating this rhythm in a patient with these symptoms.

12. d. Lead I is negative, indicating that the energy is traveling toward the negative electrode located at ∓180 degrees on the hexaxial diagram. Lead aV_F is positive, indicating that the energy is traveling toward the positive electrode located at +90 degrees. The area between +90 degrees and ∓180 degrees indicates a right axis.

13. b. Lead II has the smallest QRS complex. The lead perpendicular to lead II is lead aV_L. The QRS complex in aV_L is negative, indicating that the electric current is moving away from the positive pole. On the hexaxial diagram, the negative pole is at +150 degrees.

14. c. Lead I is positive, indicating that the energy is traveling toward the positive pole located at 0 degrees on the hexaxial diagram. Lead aV_F is also positive, indicating that the energy is flowing toward the positive pole located at +90 degrees. The area between 0 degrees and +90 degrees indicates a normal axis.

15. a. Lead aV_L has the smallest QRS complex. The lead perpendicular to lead aV_L is lead II. Lead II is positive, so the energy is traveling toward the positive pole located at +60 degrees.

16. b. Using the small block method, you'll find that the ventricular rate is 107 beats/minute. The space between the R waves takes up 14 small blocks. 1,500 ÷ 14 = 107 beats/minute.

17. b. The PR interval takes up 3 small blocks. 3 × 0.04 = 0.12 second.

18. b. The QRS complex measures 2.5 small blocks. 2.5 × 0.04 = 0.10 second.

19. c. The QT interval measures 9 small blocks. 9 × 0.04 = 0.36 second.

20. c. The delta wave indicates the preexcitation phase of Wolff-Parkinson-White syndrome.

21. b. Lead I is positive, indicating that the energy is traveling toward the positive pole located at 0 degrees on the hexaxial diagram. Lead aV$_F$ is negative, indicating that the energy is traveling away from the positive pole toward − 90 degrees. The area between 0 degrees and − 90 degrees indicates a left axis.

22. b. The QRS complex in lead V$_1$ is monophasic and positive. The QRS complex in lead V$_6$ is negative.

23. c. The QRS complex measures 5 small blocks. 5 × 0.04 = 0.20 second. The distance between two R waves is 10 small blocks. 1,500 ÷ 10 = 150 beats/minute.

24. a. The lead with the smallest QRS complex is lead aV$_R$. The lead perpendicular to lead aV$_R$ is lead III. Lead III has a negative QRS complex, indicating that energy is flowing away from the positive pole toward − 60 degrees.

25. a. The following clues point to supraventricular tachycardia. In lead V$_1$, the QRS complex is negative. In lead V$_2$, the R wave is 0.02 second, and the S wave isn't slurred or notched. The distance from the beginning of the QRS complex to the most negative point of S wave (nadir) is 0.05 second.

26. b. Adenosine has a half-life of a few minutes and takes effect within seconds. It interrupts impulse transmission in the AV node and can cause brief episodes of asystole.

27. a. The anterior wall leads V$_3$ and V$_4$ have ST-segment elevation and T-wave inversion. The lateral wall leads I and aV$_L$ have T-wave inversion, and the lateral wall leads V$_5$ and V$_6$ have ST-segment elevation plus T-wave inversion. The inferior wall leads II, III, and aV$_F$ have ST-segment elevation and T-wave inversion. These findings indicate an acute infarction in the anterior, inferior, and lateral walls.

28. b. Lead I is positive, indicating that energy is flowing toward the positive pole of lead I at 0 degrees on the hexaxial diagram. Lead aV$_F$ is negative, indicating that energy is traveling away from lead aV$_F$ toward − 90 degrees. The area between 0 degrees and − 90 degrees indicates a left axis.

29. c. A Q wave is the initial negative deflection of the QRS complex. The only leads that have an initial negative deflection are leads II, III, and aV$_F$. These Q waves are considered pathologic because they're more than 0.04 second or greater than 25% of the R-wave height.

30. b. Leads II, III, and aV$_F$ monitor the inferior wall of the left ventricle.

31. d. The right coronary artery supplies the inferior wall of the left ventricle.

32. b. Type I second-degree AV block is the only type to meet all these criteria. First-degree AV block and Type II second-degree AV block both have constant PR intervals. Third-degree AV block has regular R-R intervals.

33. c. The quadrant method indicates a left axis. The QRS complex is 0.10 second. The QRS complex configuration is qR in leads I and aV$_L$, and rS in leads II, III, and aV$_F$. These findings support left anterior hemiblock.

34. d. The deep symmetrical T-wave inversion indicates Wellens' syndrome, a critical stenosis of the proximal LAD artery.

Index

A

AAI pacemaker, 200
  ECG spikes and, 201i
Accelerated junctional rhythm,
  53i
Acebutolol, 184t
Action potential, 12
  antiarrhythmics and, 173i
Action potential curve, 14i
Acute myocardial infarction,
  97-115
  assessment findings in, 99, 101
  causes of, 98
  chest pain in, 99
  ECG changes in, 100i,
    101-103, 101i
  evaluating damage in, 101i,
    102t
  phases of, 100i, 101-102
  types of, 103-111
Adenosine, 189
Afterdepolarization, 15
Alarm, false-high-rate, troubleshooting, 38t
Amiodarone
  dosage, 186
  ECG changes and, 186
  indications for, 185
  nursing considerations for, 186
Angina, unstable, 87-95
  assessment findings in, 89
  causes of, 88-89
  chest pain in, 89
  ECG changes in, 89-91, 91i
  identifying affected vessel in,
    90-91
  monitoring patient with, 89i
  treatment of, 92-95
Angioplasty, unstable angina and,
  95
Anterior leads, 71
Anterior wall MI, 104-105
  characteristics of, 104i,
    105-106
  left bundle-branch block and,
    124
  locating damage in, 102t
  monitoring, 103i

Antiarrhythmic drugs, 171-179
  action potential and, 173i
  classification of, 172
  clearance of, 172
  distribution of, 172
  ECG changes in, 176
  risks of using, 189
  system assessment and,
    175-176
Antitachycardial pacing, 198
Aortic valve, 4-5, 7i
Apical MI, 110
  locating damage in, 102t
Arrhythmias
  causes of, 14-15
  types of, 41-63
Artifact, troubleshooting, 38t
Aspirin, unstable angina and, 95
Asynchronous pacemaker program, 197
Atenolol, 184t
Atherosclerosis, angina and, 88
Atria, 4, 7i
Atrial arrhythmias, 42, 47-51
Atrial demand-inhibiting pace-
  maker, 200, 201i
Atrial event, pacemaker evaluation
  and, 204
Atrial fibrillation, 51, 51i, 145
  assessment findings in, 145
  causes of, 145
  ECG changes in, 143i, 145
  monitoring, 144i
  treatment of, 145
Atrial flutter, 50, 50i, 143
  assessment findings in, 143,
    145
  causes of, 143
  ECG changes in, 142i, 145
  monitoring, 144i
  treatment of, 145
Atrial gallop, 99
Atrial MI, 111
Atrial rate, determining, 27
Atrial tachycardia, 48, 48i, 140
  assessment findings in, 141
  causes of, 140-141
  ECG changes in, 141-142,
    141i
  treatment of, 142
  types of, 49i

i refers to illustration; t refers to table

Atrioventricular node, 9i, 11
Atrioventricular valves, 4, 7i
Augmented limb leads, 68
    monitoring, 70i
    views of heart and, 80i
Automatic implantable cardiover-
    ter-defibrillator, 198
Automaticity
    altered, arrhythmias and, 15
    pacemaker cells and, 12
AV block, 42, 60-63
AV interval, pacemaker evaluation
    and, 204, 207
AV nodal reentry tachycardia,
    134-135
    assessment findings in, 135
    causes of, 135
    ECG changes in, 135, 137,
        137i
    monitoring, 144i
    pathophysiology of, 136i
    treatment of, 137-138
AV node, 9i, 11
AV-sequential pacemaker, 200,
    201i, 202-203
Axis deviation, causes of, 83, 85

B
Bachmann's bundle, 9i, 11
Baseline problems, troubleshoot-
    ing, 38t, 39t
Beta blockers. *See also* Class II
    antiarrhythmics.
    acute MI and, 113
    unstable angina and, 95
Bicuspid valve, 4, 7i
Bidirectional conduction, 10i
Bifascicular block, 129
    causes of, 129
    ECG changes in, 129-130,
        130i, 131i
Biphasic waveforms, 20
Bipolar limb leads, 68
    monitoring, 69i
    views of heart and, 80i
Bipolar pacing system, 194i
Box method, atrial rate and, 27
Bradycardia, blood flow and, 6
Bretylium
    dosage, 186

Bretylium *(continued)*
    ECG changes and, 187
    indications for, 186
    nursing considerations for, 187
Bundle-branch block, 118
    left, 118, 120i, 122, 124, 125i
    right, 118, 120i, 122-124,
        123i
Bundle branches, 9i, 11
Bundle of His, 9i, 11
Burst pacing, 48

C
CAD. *See* Coronary artery disease,
    risk factors for.
Calcium channel blockers. *See
    also* Class IV antiarrhythmics.
    acute MI and, 114
    unstable angina and, 95
Calcium deficiency. *See* Hypocal-
    cemia.
Calcium imbalances, 160-164
Calipers method, rhythm deter-
    mination and, 26i
Cardiac catheterization, 113
Cardiac chambers, 4, 7i
Cardiac enzyme analysis, 111
Cardiac rehabilitation, 115
Cardiac veins, 6, 8i
Cardiovascular system
    anatomy of, 4-6, 5i, 7-9i
    antiarrhythmic therapy and,
        175
    physiology of, 6, 11-12, 13i,
        14, 14i
Celiprolol, 184t
Chest pain
    in acute MI, 99
    in angina, 89
Chest X-ray, 111-112
Chordae tendineae, 4, 7i
Circus movement tachycardia,
    138
    causes of, 138-139
    ECG changes in, 139, 140i
    monitoring, 144i
    pathophysiology of, 138i
    significance of, 139
    treatment of, 139
Circus reentry, 10i, 15

Class IA antiarrhythmics, 176-179
  action of, 176
  ECG changes and, 176, 177i
  major drugs used as, 176-179
Class I antiarrhythmics, 176-183.
    See also specific categories.
  action potential and, 173i
Class IB antiarrhythmics, 180-182
  action of, 180
  ECG changes and, 180, 180i
  major drugs used as, 180-182
Class IC antiarrhythmics, 182-183
  action of, 182
  ECG changes and, 182, 183i
  major drugs used as, 182-183
Class II antiarrhythmics, 183-185
  action potential and, 173i
  dosage, 184t
  ECG changes and, 184-185,
      185i
  nursing considerations for, 185
  types of, 183-184
Class III antiarrhythmics, 185-187
  action of, 185
  action potential and, 173i
  ECG changes and, 186i
  major drugs used as, 185-187
Class IV antiarrhythmics, 187-189
  action of, 187
  action potential and, 173i
  ECG changes and, 188i
  major drugs used as, 187-189
Collateral circulation, 6
Complete heart block, 63, 63i
Conduction system, 6, 9i, 11
Coronary artery bypass graft sur-
    gery
  acute MI and, 115
  unstable angina and, 95
Coronary artery disease, risk fac-
    tors for, 98
Coronary blood flow, 5-6, 8i
Coronary vasospasm, angina and,
    88-89

D
DDD pacemaker, 203-204
  ECG spikes and, 202i
DDD pacing mode, 198
Deflections, waveform, 20, 20i
Degree method, electrical axis
    determination and, 83, 84i

Delta wave, 139i
Depolarization-repolarization,
    phases of, 12, 13i, 14, 14i,
    15
Diabetes mellitus, CAD and, 98
Diaphragmatic pacing, 207t
Diastole, coronary artery blood
    flow and, 6
Diltiazem, 188
Disopyramide
  dosage, 179
  ECG changes and, 179
  indications for, 179
  nursing considerations for, 179
  pharmacodynamics of, 179
Drug-induced arrhythmias, 172.
    See also Proarrhythmias.
Dual-chamber pacemakers, 200,
    201-202i, 202-204
  ECG spikes and, 201-202i
DVI pacemaker, 200, 202-203
  ECG spikes and, 201i

E
ECG. *See* Electrocardiography *and*
    Electrocardiograms, analyz-
    ing.
ECG changes
  in acute MI, 100i, 101-103,
      101i
  adenosine and, 189
  amiodarone and, 186
  antiarrhythmic drugs and, 176
  in atrial fibrillation, 143i, 145
  in atrial flutter, 142i, 145
  in atrial tachycardia, 141-142,
      141i
  in AV nodal reentry tachycar-
      dia, 135, 137, 137i
  beta blockers and, 183-185,
      185i
  in bifascicular block, 129-130,
      130i, 131i
  bretylium and, 187
  in circus movement tachycar-
      dia, 139, 140i
  class IA antiarrhythmics and,
      176, 177i
  class IB antiarrhythmics and,
      180, 180i
  class IC antiarrhythmics and,
      182, 183i

i refers to illustration; t refers to table

ECG changes *(continued)*
    class II antiarrhythmics and,
        184-185, 185i
    class III antiarrhythmics and,
        186i
    class IV antiarrhythmics and,
        188i
    diltiazem and, 188
    disopyramide and, 179
    in heart blocks, 122
    in hypercalcemia, 161, 162i
    in hyperkalemia, 156-158,
        157i
    in hypermagnesemia, 164-165,
        165i
    in hypocalcemia, 163, 163i
    in hypokalemia, 159-160, 159i
    in hypomagnesemia, 167
    in left anterior hemiblock,
        125-127, 126i
    in left bundle-branch block,
        124, 125i
    in left posterior hemiblock,
        127i, 129
    in narrow QRS-complex tachy-
        cardias, 134, 135i
    nifedipine and, 189
    pacemakers and, 192
    procainamide and, 179
    quinidine and, 177, 178i
    in right bundle-branch block,
        123-124, 123i
    sotalol and, 187
    in supraventricular rhythms,
        151i, 152-153
    in unstable angina, 89-91, 91i
    in ventricular tachycardia,
        148-149i, 149-152
    verapamil and, 187-188
ECG grid, 21, 21i
ECG strip, 21-22, 21i
Echocardiography, 112
Electrical axis
    determination of, 81, 82i, 83
    deviation, causes of, 83, 85
    direction of, 80-81, 82i, 83
Electrical interference, 76-77
    troubleshooting, 38t
Electrical interference, trouble-
    shooting, 38t
Electrocardiograms, analyzing,
    27-29

Electrocardiography, 20-22
Electrode tips, 193
Electrolyte disturbances, 155-167
Electrophysiology, 11-12, 13i, 14,
    14i
Encainide, 182-183
Endocardial lead placement, 193,
    195i
Endocardium, 4
Epicardium, 4
Escape beat, 11
Escape rhythms, 11
Excitability, nonpacemaker cells
    and, 12

F

Failure to capture, 205t
Failure to pace, 205t
Failure to sense, 206t
First-degree AV block, 60, 60i
First-pass studies, 113
Five-leadwire system, 32-33
    lead placement in, 32i, 34i
Flecainide, 182
Focal reentry, 15
Fuzzy baseline, troubleshooting,
    39t

G

Gastrointestinal system, antiar-
    rhythmic therapy and, 176
Gated heart studies, 112-113
Genetic factors, CAD and, 98

H

Hardwire monitoring, 32-33
Heart, anatomy of, 4-6, 5i
Heart blocks, 117-131
    assessment findings in, 118
    causes of, 118
    ECG changes in, 122
    treatment of, 131
    types of, 122
Heart murmur, acute MI and, 99
Hexaxial reference system, 80-81,
    81i, 82i, 83
Hypercalcemia, 160
    assessment findings in,
        160-161
    causes of, 160
    ECG changes in, 161, 162i
    treatment of, 161-162

i refers to illustration; t refers to table

Hyperkalemia, 156
  assessment findings in, 156
  causes of, 156
  ECG changes in, 156-158,
    157i
  monitoring patient with, 158i
  renal failure and, 156
  treatment of, 158
Hyperlipidemia, CAD and, 98
Hypermagnesemia, 164
  assessment findings in, 164
  causes of, 164
  ECG changes in, 164-165,
    165i
  treatment of, 165
Hypertension, CAD and, 98
Hypocalcemia, 162
  assessment findings in,
    162-163
  causes of, 162
  ECG changes in, 163, 163i
  treatment of, 163-164
Hypokalemia, 158
  assessment findings in,
    158-159
  causes of, 158
  digoxin and, 160
  ECG changes in, 159-160,
    159i
  mild vs. severe, 161i
  treatment of, 160
Hypomagnesemia, 165-166
  assessment findings in, 167
  causes of, 166-167
  ECG changes in, 167
  treatment of, 167

I
Idioventricular rhythm, 59, 59i
Inferior leads, 71
Inferior wall MI, 106
  characteristics of, 106, 108i
  left anterior hemiblock and,
    127
  locating damage in, 102t
  monitoring, 103i
Instant-to-instant vectors, 80
Internodal tracts, 9i, 11
Interventricular conduction block.
    See Heart blocks.
Intra-aortic balloon pump, 115

Isoelectric deflection, 20
Isoelectric line, 20
  ECG and, 12

JK
J point, 22i, 24
J-point depression, 90i
Junctional arrhythmias, 42, 52-54
Junctional rhythm, 52, 52i
  types of, 53i
Junctional tachycardia, 53i

L
Labetalol, 184t
Lateral leads, 71
Lateral wall MI, 106
  characteristics of, 106, 107i
  locating damage in, 102t
  monitoring, 103i
Lead I, 37
Lead II, 37
Lead MCL$_1$, 35i, 36
Leads, 20-21
Leads MCL$_2$ to MCL$_6$, 35i, 36
Leads V$_2$ and V$_3$, 37
Leads V$_4$ and V$_5$, 37
Lead V$_1$, 37
Left anterior hemiblock, 121i,
    124-125
  causes of, 125
  ECG changes in, 125-127,
    126i
  inferior wall MI and, 127
  monitoring patient with, 128i
Left axis deviation, 83, 85
Left bundle-branch block, 120i,
    124
  anterior wall MI and, 124
  causes of, 124
  ECG changes in, 124, 125i
  monitoring patient with, 128i
Left main coronary artery disease,
    91, 94i
Left posterior hemiblock, 121i,
    129
  causes of, 129
  ECG changes in, 127i, 129
  monitoring patient with, 128i
Lewis lead, 35i, 37
Lidocaine, 180

Limb leads, 68
   monitoring, 69i, 70i
   views of heart and, 80i

M
Magnesium deficiency. *See* Hypo-
   magnesemia.
Magnesium imbalances, 164-167
Magnetic resonance imaging, 112
Membrane potential, 12
Metoprolol, 184t
Mexiletine, 180-181
MI. *See* Acute myocardial infarc-
   tion.
Mitral valve, 4, 7i
M-mode echocardiography, 112
Mobitz I AV block, 61, 61i
Mobitz II AV block, 62, 62i
Monitoring
   hardwire, 32-33
   lead selection in, 33, 34i, 35i
   simultaneous dual, 36i
   telemetry, 33
   troubleshooting problems in,
      38-39t
Moricizine, 181
Morphine sulfate, 113
MUGA scanning, 113
Multifocal atrial tachycardia, 49i
Multiple-gated acquisition scans,
   113
Myocardium, 4, 7i

N
Nadolol, 184t
Narrow QRS-complex tachycar-
   dias, 134-145
   ECG changes in, 134, 135i
   monitoring, 144i
   types of, 134-145
NBG coding system, 197-198
Negative deflection, 20, 20i
Nervous system, antiarrhythmic
   therapy and, 176
Nifedipine, 189
Nitrates, unstable angina and,
   94-95
Nitroglycerin, 113
Noninvasive transcutaneous car-
   diac pacing, 195, 197
Nonpacemaker cells, 12, 14i

Normal sinus rhythm, 42, 42i
Nuclear imaging, 112-113
Nuclear wall motion studies,
   112-113

O
Obesity, CAD and, 98
Oversensing, 206t
Oxprenolol, 184t

P
Pacemaker cells, automaticity
   and, 12, 15
Pacemakers, 191-207
   codes for, 197-198
   components of, 192-193
   ECG characteristics of, 192
   evaluating function of, 204,
      205-207t, 207
   indications for, 192
   monitoring patients with, 204i
   placement of, 193, 195, 195i,
      197
   reprogramming, 199i
   troubleshooting problems with,
      205-207t
   types of, 198-200, 202-204
Pacing at altered rate, 207t
Pacing leads, 193, 194i
Paper-pencil method, rhythm determination and, 26i
Papillary muscles, 4, 7i
Paroxysmal atrial tachycardia, 49i,
   140
Percutaneous transluminal coronary angioplasty, 115
Pericardial friction rub, 99, 101
Pericardium, 4
Permanent pacemaker, lead
   placement for, 193, 195i
Phenytoin as antiarrhythmic,
   181-182
Pindolol, 184t
Planes, 20
Platelet aggregation, 88
   angina and, 88
   aspirin and, 95
Positive deflection, 20
Posterior wall MI, 108
   characteristics of, 108-109,
      110i, 111i
   locating damage in, 102t

i refers to illustration; t refers to table

Potassium deficiency. *See* Hypokalemia.
Potassium imbalances, 156-160
P-P interval, 26i, 27
Precordial leads, 68, 71
  placement of, 71i
Premature atrial contractions, 47,
  47i
Premature junctional contractions,
  54, 54i
Premature ventricular contrac-
  tions, 55, 55i
PR interval, 23-24, 28
Proarrhythmias, 172
  depiction of, on action poten-
    tial curve, 174i
  development of, 175i
  risk factors for, 173
Procainamide
  dosage, 177
  ECG changes and, 179
  indications for, 177
  nursing considerations for, 179
  pharmacodynamics of, 177-179
Propafenone, 183
Propranolol, 184t
P-synchronous pacing, 203
Pulmonary valve, 4-5, 7i
Pulse generator, 193
Purkinje fibers, 9i, 11
P wave, 22i, 23, 28i

Q
QRS complex, 24, 28, 28i, 29i
QT interval, 25, 28-29
Quadrant method, electrical axis
  determination and, 81, 82i,
  83
Quinidine
  dosage, 177
  ECG changes and, 177
  indications for, 176-177
  nursing considerations for, 177
  toxicity, 178i
Q wave, 22i, 24
  pathologic, 102-103

R
Reentry
  circus, 10i, 15
  focal, 15

Refractory period, 12, 14i, 15
Renal failure, hyperkalemia and,
  156
Repolarization, 12. *See also* Depo-
  larization-repolarization,
  phases of.
Reprogramming pacemaker, 199i
Respiratory system, antiarrhyth-
  mic therapy and, 175
Resting membrane potential, 12
Retrograde conduction, 15
Rhythm, determination of, 26i
Rhythm strip, obtaining, 37
Right axis deviation, 83, 85
Right bundle-branch block, 120i,
  122
  causes of, 122-123
  ECG changes in, 123-124,
    123i
  monitoring patient with, 128i
Right ventricular MI, 106
  characteristics of, 107, 109i
R-on-T phenomenon, 57i
R-R interval, 25, 26i, 27
R wave, 22i, 24

S
SA node, 9i, 11
Second-degree AV block
  atrial tachycardia and, 49i
  Type I, 61, 61i
  Type II, 62, 62i
Sedentary life-style, CAD and, 98
Semilunar valves, 4, 7i
Septal wall MI, 106
  characteristics of, 105, 106
  locating damage in, 102t
Signal-average ECG, 76, 77
Signals, weak, troubleshooting,
  38t
Silent ischemia, 90
Simultaneous dual monitoring,
  36i
Single-chamber pacemakers, 200
  ECG spikes and, 201i
Single-lead monitoring, 31-39
Sinoatrial node, 9i, 11
Sinus arrest, 46, 46i
Sinus arrhythmia, 43, 43i
Sinus arrhythmias, 42, 43-46
Sinus bradycardia, 44, 44i

i refers to illustration; t refers to table

Sinus pause, 46
Sinus tachycardia, 45, 45i
Smoking, CAD and, 98
Sodium-potassium pump, 13i, 14
Sotalol
    as class II antiarrhythmic, 184t
    as class III antiarrhythmic, 187
Sternal lead, 35i, 37
Stimulation threshold, testing, 196i
Stress, CAD and, 98
ST segment, 24-25
ST-segment depression, 90i
ST-segment monitoring, 101i
Subendocardial MI, 109-110
Supraventricular rhythms, 152
    assessment findings in, 152
    ECG changes in, 151i, 152-153
    pathophysiology of, 150i
    treatment of, 153
S wave, 22i, 24
Synchronous pacemaker program, 197
Systole, coronary artery blood flow and, 6

T
Tachycardia, 133-153
    blood flow and, 6
    narrow QRS-complex, 134-145
    wide QRS-complex, 145-153
Ta wave, 23
Technetium scanning, 112
Telemetry, 33
    lead placement in, 34i
Temporary pacemaker
    stimulation threshold and, 196i
    transcutaneous lead placement for, 195, 197
    transmediastinal lead placement for, 193, 195
    transthoracic lead placement for, 195
    transvenous lead placement for, 195
Thallium imaging, 112
Third-degree AV block, 63, 63i
Three leadwire system, 33
    lead placement in, 33i, 34i
Thrombolytic therapy, 114
Thrombosis, angina and, 88

Times ten method, atrial rate and, 27
Timolol, 184t
Tocainide, 181
Torsades de pointes, 57i, 147i
Tp wave, 23
Transcutaneous cardiac pacing, 195, 197
Transcutaneous placement, temporary pacemaker and, 195, 197
Transmediastinal placement, temporary pacemaker and, 193, 195
Transthoracic placement, temporary pacemaker and, 195
Transvenous placement, temporary pacemaker and, 195
Tricuspid valve, 4, 7i
Trifascicular block, 130-131. See also Complete heart block.
Triggered activity, 15
T wave, 22i, 24, 25
Twelve-lead ECG, 20-21, 67-77. See also Electrocardiograms, analyzing.
    components of, 68, 69i, 70i, 71, 71i
    electrical interference and, 76-77
    interpreting, 75-76, 75i
    recording, 72-74i
Two-dimensional echocardiography, 112

U
Ultrasound imaging, 112
Unidirectional conduction, 10i
Unipolar pacing system, 194i
U wave, 22i, 25-26

V
VA interval, pacemaker evaluation and, 207
Valves, 4-5, 7i
VAT pacing mode, 197-198
VDD pacemaker, 203
    ECG spikes and, 202i
VDD pacing mode, 198
Vectors, instant-to-instant, 80
Ventricles, 4, 7i

i refers to illustration; t refers to table

Ventricular activation
  abnormal, 118, 120-121i
  normal, 118, 119i
Ventricular arrhythmias, 42,
    55-59
Ventricular event, pacemaker eval-
    uation and, 207
Ventricular fibrillation, 58, 58i
Ventricular tachycardia, 56, 56i,
    147
  assessment findings in,
    147-149
  ECG changes in, 148-149i,
    149-152
  treatment of, 153
  variations of, 57i
Verapamil
  dosage, 187
  ECG changes and, 187-188
  indications for, 187
  nursing considerations for, 188
  pharmacodynamics of, 187
VOO pacing mode, 198
VVI pacemaker, 200
  ECG spikes and, 201i
VVI pacing mode, 198

WXYZ
Wandering baseline, troubleshoot-
    ing, 38t
Waveforms
  absence of, 39t
  components of, 22-26, 22i
  deflections of, 20, 20i
  interference with, 38t
Wellens syndrome, 89i, 91
  ECG changes in, 91, 92i
Wenckebach AV block, 61, 61i
Wide QRS-complex tachycardias,
    145-153
  monitoring, 152i
  pathophysiology of, 146i
  treatment of, 153
  types of, 146-153
Wireless monitoring, 33
Wolff-Parkinson-White syndrome,
    139i